Intermittent Fasting For Body and Mind

Weight Loss is Just the Tip of the Iceberg

By Peter Hardwood

© **Copyright 2019 - All rights reserved.**

The content contained within this book may not be reproduced, duplicated or transmitted without direct written permission from the author or the publisher.

Under no circumstances will any blame or legal responsibility be held against the publisher, or author, for any damages, reparation, or monetary loss due to the information contained within this book. Either directly or indirectly.

Legal Notice:

This book is copyright protected. This book is only for personal use. You cannot amend, distribute, sell, use, quote or paraphrase any part, or the content within this book, without the consent of the author or publisher.

Disclaimer Notice:

Please note the information contained within this document is for educational and entertainment purposes only. All effort has been executed to present accurate, up to date, and reliable, complete information. No warranties of any kind are declared or implied. Readers acknowledge that the author is not engaging in the rendering of legal, financial, medical or professional advice. The content within this book has been derived from various sources. Please consult a licensed professional before attempting any techniques outlined in this book.

By reading this document, the reader agrees that under no circumstances is the author responsible for any losses, direct or indirect, which are incurred as a result of the use of information contained within this document, including, but not limited to, — errors, omissions, or inaccuracies.

Table of Contents

Introduction 4
Chapter 1: Causes of Weight Gain and Obesity 7
Chapter 2: Signs of Bad Diets and Lifestyles 15
Chapter 3: What is Fasting? 24
Chapter 4: Myths about Intermittent Fasting 31
Chapter 5: What Happens to the Body During a Fast? 41
Chapter 6: Different Fasting Techniques 50
Chapter 7: What Comes with Fasting 63
Chapter 8: How to Take the First Steps .. 85
Chapter 9: The Potential Downsides of Intermittent Fasting 139
Conclusion 147

Introduction

Our health is one of the most important aspects of our lives that we have. There are so many things that we need to watch out for, and we assume that it is impossible to take care of it all, and may lament that we are likely to deal with one health condition or another with nothing we can do to fix it. But this just isn't true. In fact, a simple eating protocol, known as intermittent fasting, will be just the ticket you need to help improve every aspect of your health, and it is so much easier than you may think!

In this guidebook, we are going to explore a lot of the different aspects that comes with an intermittent fast, and how you can use this to your advantage to improve your health. With so many different protocols to choose from, it makes sense that many people run to this method to help them lose weight and improve their health in many ways.

While many people choose to go on an intermittent fast to lose weight, and this is certainly an effective way for you to lose weight if needed, there is so much more that you are able to benefit from with a fast, that it would be a shame to exclude all of them just for weight loss. As we will explore in this guidebook, almost every aspect of your health, from your blood pressure to your high blood sugars to your mental clarity and more can be improved, simply by going on an intermittent fast and limiting your eating window.

Seems too good to be true? It really isn't. By learning how to limit your eating window either daily or throughout the week, you are allowing the body to have time to heal itself, and even speed up the metabolism as you give the body a break from all of that bad food. If you are able to combine it together with a healthy diet, which is highly encouraged on this eating plan, you will be able to not only lose the weight that you want, but improve your health and feel better in so many ways.

As we will discuss and show in this guidebook, intermittent fasting is an easy process to follow, and there are many choices that you can make when it comes to working with this eating plan. This makes it perfect for you to really fit this into your schedule, which increases your chances of all the health benefits that come from intermittent fasting.

When you are ready to learn more about how intermittent fasting works, and what you can do to improve your health and help with your blood pressure, mental clarity, blood sugar levels, and weight loss, make sure to check out this guidebook to help you get started.

Chapter 1: Causes of Weight Gain and Obesity

Obesity is known as a serious and chronic disease that is going to negatively affect many different parts of your body. People who are considered obese or overweight are going to have a higher risk when it comes to developing serious conditions including bone and joint diseases, type 2 diabetes, heart disease, pain, lack of mobility, and more.

The obesity epidemic is growing so much in the United States. According to the U.S. Surgeon General, it is believed that 35 percent of women and 31 percent of men are considered seriously overweight. In addition, 15 percent of children between the ages of six and 19 in this country are considered overweight too. This shows us that the obesity epidemic is not just about adults any longer. It is also going to be a problem that younger and younger children are going to deal with as well.

As the obesity epidemic starts to spread, public health officials are going to warn that the results of physical activity, along with a poor diet, are going to catch up to tobacco when it comes to how much they are going to threaten our health. Learning how to take care of your health and lower the amount of weight that you are carrying around due to inactivity and poor diet choices, is one of the best ways to fight the many diseases that are going to be associated with obesity and extra weight.

Consequences of obesity

Obesity is definitely a problem that a lot of people are starting to face, not only in the United States but in other developed countries as well. Our hectic lifestyles, the poor food choices, and the fact that many jobs do not have us up and moving around often are all contributing to this kind of weight gain.

But allowing this to be an excuse for us and not dealing with it is going to cause us a lot of issues in the long run. In fact, there is a long laundry list of consequences that are going to happen when we are dealing with obesity, and when we allow it to stick around for the long term. Some of the major consequences that we are able to face when we are dealing with obesity will include:

Metabolic syndrome

The first consequence of obesity that we are going to take a look at is known as metabolic syndrome. This is going to be more of an umbrella term that is going to explore many different issues such as:

High blood pressure

High blood sugar levels even when the person is in a fasting state
Low levels of HDL cholesterol (or the good kind) in the blood
High levels of triglycerides in the blood
Increased circumference around the waist.

Obesity is going to be the underlying cause of many of these disorders, and the more weight that the individual is carrying around, the more likely it is that they are also dealing with this condition along the way. Being able to control your weight and get it down to healthier levels is critical to ensuring that you are going to be able to prevent and even heal metabolic syndrome.

Hypertension

Many of the foods that those who are obese consume are going to be prone to increased levels of hypertension throughout the body. The combination of fats, sodium, cholesterol, and even sugars and carbs are going to contribute to higher blood pressure levels. Add in that there is going to be a lot of in activities that don't help to make the heart stronger, and it is no wonder that those who are obese are also going to deal with issues of higher heart rates.

Hormonal changes

There are also going to be some changes in your hormones when you gain weight and become obese. There are a number of hormones that we need to take a look at and figure out how they are going to be influenced when we see some changes in our levels of hormones.

First, we are going to look at obesity and leptin. This hormone is going to be produced by the fat cells of the body before being released into the blood. Leptin is going to reduce our appetite by acting on certain parts of the brain to help reduce the urge we have to eat. It is also going to have some control in managing how we store fat on the body. Since leptin is going to be produced by fat, when someone is obese, they are going to have higher levels of leptin. But the problem comes when these people are not sensitive to leptin and even though there is more of it in the body, they are not going to respond to it well, and will not know when they are full or how to control their appetites.

Then there is going to be insulin. This is an important hormone to follow when it comes to regulating carbs in the body and even metabolizing the fats. Insulin is going to stimulate glucose uptake from the blood in tissues such as the liver and muscles. It is important because it makes sure that the cells of the body are getting the energy that they need. But when someone is obese, these signals from insulin are going to get lost, and it becomes hard to regular and controls the levels of glucose in the body. If this is not taken care of, it is going to result in the person dealing with metabolic syndrome and type 2 diabetes.

Obesity is able to affect the growth hormones as well. The pituitary gland in the brain is going to produce this hormone, which is going to help influence the height of a person and will help to build up muscles and bones in the body as well. Growth hormones are also there in order to affect our metabolism and how fast it is going to be able to burn through the foods that we eat. According to some research, it has been found that the growth hormone levels in people who are obese are going to be lower compared to those who are in their normal weight levels.

Pain

Obesity and pain are going to present us with a very serious public health concern for all of society. There is a strong amount of evidence that suggests that obesity is going to be common in many conditions of chronic pain, and complaints of pain are going to be very common in those who are obese.

There are a number of reasons that this could be happening. The added weight to the person is going to put more pressure on the bones and joints than it does for normal people. This makes it more painful just to do normal activities that others may not find as a problem. These individuals may be less likely to move around and do physical activity, causing them to lose muscle mass and to get stiff from sitting still. Both of these can result in some pain when the person decides to get up and move.

Cholesterol levels that are elevated

Elevated cholesterol levels are going to be a bad thing for your heart health. It is going to make it difficult for you to really keep your heart health strong, and it can cause your blood pressure to rise, the heart to pump harder, and more issues along the way. This is something that you need to be able to get under control if you want to be able to keep your health up and running.

When you eat foods that are full of the wrong kinds of fats, along with a lot of cholesterol as well, you may find that it is really hard to keep your cholesterol levels in check. This is going to make it so that particles start to build up in the bloodstream and stick to the arteries and more. Then they start to stick to one another. This causes issues because it limits the amount of room in the arteries for the blood to pump through, and causes you to put too much pressure on the arteries and the heart.

This is more likely to happen when you are obese because you are eating foods that are unhealthy and bad for you. Foods that are high in fats, high in calories, and will contribute you to being obese are ones that are going to elevate your cholesterol levels. When you change up your lifestyle and your diet plan and learn how to be more active, you will find that you can naturally lower your cholesterol levels in the process.

There are a lot of consequences that can happen when you are dealing with obesity, and it is important to be able to limit it as much as possible. When you are able to find ways to really work on controlling your diet, adding in some more physical activity to your life, and taking control over your health, you will find that it is easier for you to avoid the consequences that come with the obesity epidemic in America.

Chapter 2: Signs of Bad Diets and Lifestyles

The leading cause of obesity, no matter what kind of genetics you have or how fast your metabolism is going or anything else, is going to be that you eat a poor diet and that you do not get up and move enough. You can try to blame the other stuff all that you want, but for most people, these are just going to be some side issues that make the situation worse, but not the main event to why they are dealing with obesity.

If you are able to get your diet and your lifestyle under control, you will find that you will be able to lose quite a bit of weight and it is going to be easier for you to maintain your health and feel you're very best. Let's take a look at how a poor diet and limited physical activity, along with other poor lifestyle choices, are the main reason that you are dealing with obesity and some of the bad health conditions that come with it.
Bad eating habits are the problem

The main problem that comes with obesity is the idea of bad eating habits. Being physically active is an important thing to focus on as well, but you will find that if you are able to get your eating style and diet down, you have won a good 80 percent of the battle along the way. The foods that you eat, along with the times you choose to eat those foods (as we will discuss a bit later), are going to make a world of difference with the weight that you are and any weight loss that you are going to try to do as well.

Many American families are not eating the way that they should. They spend too much time eating out, picking out meals that are fast and from the freezer section, and enjoying a lot of baked goods from the store. Making a home-cooked meal takes a lot of time, and whether they don't feel like doing it or just don't have the time, this is a lot of work for many people.

It is common to see way too many calories, coupled with too many fats, carbs, sugars, sodium and more, packed into the daily lifestyle of most Americans. And since they are not being active enough to burn off these calories by any stretch of the imagination, it is no wonder that they are just causing themselves to gain weight and get sicker over time.

Instead of eating these bad foods, it is time to make some changes and see if you are able to eat foods that are so much better for you. Our bodies are crying out for foods that are healthy and wholesome, ones that are going to give us a lot of the nutrients that we need, without making us take on too many calories in the process.

There are a lot of different foods that you can start implementing into your diet to help you stay healthy and to actually provide your body with the nutrients that it so desperately needs. First, stick with the produce. Lots of healthy and wholesome produce is going to fill you up, can taste so good, and will provide you with a lot of the nutrients that you need to be as healthy as possible. Try to add in a lot of variety so you can mix it up and never get bored in the process.

Next is the lean meats. This will provide you with the protein that you need to build up those muscles again and to make sure that you are not going to feel as much pain or discomfort when you start working out again. Going with options like turkey, chicken, steak, beef, and fish can be a great way to increase your health while losing weight.

Carbs are not all bad, but you do need to be mindful of how many and how much you are consuming when it is time to fight off the obesity that you are dealing with. You want to go with options that are whole wheat or whole grain rather than any that are found in sweets or the ones that are considered processed.

Healthy sources of dairy products like yogurt, milk cheese, sour cream, cottage cheese, and more can really help as well. These will make sure that your bones and your joints are getting the nutrients that they need to stay strong so that you no longer feel any more pain or discomfort from them along the way.

So, if you have started to notice that you are dealing with a lot of brain fog on a regular basis, or you are feeling tired, sluggish, irritated, bloated, or a lot of bad health conditions are starting to appear when you visit the doctor, then it is time for you to make some changes to your diet and lifestyle. The tips above will help you with the diet portion of the plan. And learning how to change up your lifestyle is as easy as adding in some more physical activity to your day.

What about lifestyle?

While the diet that we follow is a big determinant in how much obesity is going to affect us or not, it is not the only thing that we have to consider. The kind of lifestyle that we follow is going to make a difference as well. If we spend most of the day doing nothing and not moving around all that much, then we are just contributing to the issue at hand.

Think about how much the average American moves around during the day. They may get up early and get ready for the day. Next, they sit in their car on the way to work, which could last for an hour or more each way. They get to work and sit down at an office all day, doing computer work or phone work or something else that doesn't get them up and moving much at all. Then they get back into the car and drive another hour or more to get home.

By this point, they are mentally exhausted, even though they did not move around much at all. They will often get a few things done, and then sit down to eat a meal, play games or watch a show on TV before going to bed. There may be a few days that are exceptions to this, but for the most part, Americans are not getting up and doing the moving that they need to in order to help their bodies stay as strong as possible.

And this is turning into a big problem. When you are sitting and not doing as many movements on a regular basis, you are not burning through the number of calories that you should during that time. When you add to the mix the fact that you are eating a lot of foods that are high in calories and bad for you, it is a recipe for disaster all around.

Where did we learn these bad habits?

The next thing that we need to take a look at here is the idea of where we are forming these bad habits. In reality, we are getting them from the world around us. It is from our parents from our friends, from our coworkers, from TV and so much more.

We are in a culture that is not really for our best health. We are told that we need to work long hours, and that usually means in an area where we are not allowed to get up and move often or where we don't have time to work out when we get home. We are told that we need to go out to eat a bunch, or maybe we just don't have the time to work on making a good home-cooked meals the way that we should. And this results in us eating a bunch of junk that is not all that good for us.

Add to that the fact that it seems there are so many medications out there that can be the quick fix to any disease that we may encounter, and it is no wonder that we are comfortable with these bad habits. We may know that they are not good for us, but the things that are good for us are harder to do and are not all that much fun. Being able to do what we want, or what we have time for, is sometimes the best option. And that is something we have learned from a young age onward.

How we get sicker following this diet

The longer that we are dealing with these bad health habits and eating habits, the worse it is going to get for us. We are just going to continue making ourselves sicker over time unless we are able to get our diets and our lifestyles under control and learn how to eat when we are hungry, avoid food when we are not, and actually see it as something that is meant to keep us alive, not something that we are going to be out of in two seconds and we have to eat as much as possible all day long.

Fighting against some of our hormonal changes, our genetics, and even some of our evolution is not going to be an easy task. But it is something that we need to do if we want to improve our health. It is going to take some work, but otherwise, our health is going to just keep deteriorating.

Many of us are in denial. We assume that we are not so bad and that it is going to be just fine if we keep going the way that we are. We may think it is just a few pounds, or that this is just the way that the weight goes as we get older and start having less metabolism or we end up not having as much free time and energy as we did in the past.

But then the weight just keeps piling on. And then we hear about the first health condition that we need to worry about. Maybe it is prediabetes or heart troubles or high blood pressure or something else. We know that this is a bad thing, but we brush it away not wanting to deal with it. We assume that it is just a fluke, that everyone in our family has that condition so it is not that big of a deal, or that we are going to be able to take it down without too much of a fight.

The problem is that even with this health concern, we may not be thinking harshly enough about it to make the changes that are needed. We choose to continue with the regular lifestyle that we have been on, and over time, the health conditions that we have and are dealing with just keep adding up. Before we know it, we have a laundry list of things that are wrong with us, and our medicine cabinets look like we are a pharmacist.

It doesn't have to be this way. We are not stuck this way, and it doesn't have to get this bad. With some healthier eating choices and a more active lifestyle, you will find that it is definitely possible to take back the control over your health that you want and to prevent yourself from getting sicker. But being in denial about it and assuming that it is not a big deal, is not going to help you. Facing your bad health decisions and figuring out what you are able to do about it right here and now is the best way to get in your best health yet.

Chapter 3: What is Fasting?

When we hear about fasting, we assume that this is a very bad thing. We worry that we are going to make ourselves sick when we go on a fast, or that we are going to be doing some really bad damage to the body that we will not be able to fix no matter how hard we try. We have been told for years that the best way to stay healthy is to eat a bunch of small meals throughout the day, in the hopes that we will keep the metabolism burning and that we will get more weight loss as a result.

But fasting is not the mean villain that it has been painted out to be. In fact, fasting is going to be a really powerful tool that you can use in order to improve your health and help you to see the results that you just can't get with other methods. Fasting has been around for thousands of years and is a method that cultures and religions all of the world have done to fight against tyranny, help them to prepare for something, and even to cleanse. Why would fasting all of a sudden be something that we need to shy away from and be worried about all of the time?

The history of fasting

There isn't necessarily a beginning point when it comes to fasting because it is believed that there were fasts all throughout humankind. Every other animal in this world will fast even in our modern times in order to deal with times when they are sick or when they are under stress. And sometimes, this fasting can happen just because we feel uneasy and like we shouldn't eat. It is actually a natural tendency to work with, whether we are human or animal, to seek out time to rest, to balance ourselves, and even to conserve some energy in the process.

Fasting is something that has been done all throughout time, and in fact, it is often one of the methods that have been used throughout time as a way to heal the body naturally without a lot of medications and other harsh methods. The early healers, thinkers, and philosophers were not scared to use fasting to help them be healthy and to help with healing others. In fact, many names that we all know like Socrates, Galen, Aristotle, Plato, and Hippocrates would praise the benefits that came with fasting.

To take this a bit further, Paracelsus, one of the three fathers of Western medicine as we know and love it today, is quoted as saying "Fasting is the greatest remedy, the physician within." Isn't it amazing to think that we have a method that can allow us to heal ourselves, and all that it takes, for many of the ailments that we deal with, is some time to abstain from food? Early healing arts already knew about the powerful healing and rejuvenation that we are able to get from fasting, but for some reason, the modern medical and healing world seems to be a bit behind with these ideas.

In addition to many of the early thinkers and healers working with fasting, it was also common that a lot of the bigger spiritual groups and religious groups would use fasting as part of their ceremonies and rites. This was often going to occur during the spring and then again during the fall, and it would be encouraged individually during other times of the year as well. Today, it is known that every major religion is going to practice some kind of fasting as a way to benefit the spirit in the process.

Think of all the religions of the world who are going to rely on some form of fasting at one point or another. North American Indian tribes, Hinduism, tribes of the South, Buddhism, Islam, Gnosticism, Judaism, and Christianity are all going to use one form or another of fasting within them. Whether this fasting is going to be used to help with sacrifice, mourning, penance, spiritual vision, or a way to help purify the soul, all of these religions are going to include some kind of fasting inside of them.

Many faiths are not just going to recommend that people fast on occasion. They are going to prescribe to regular fasting to prevent or to break the habits of gluttony. Some of the religious groups that are most noted for continuing this tradition of fasting in the United States will include the Jews, Lutherans, Roman Catholics, and Episcopalians.

These are major religions that are found all throughout the world and have been around for many years now. And all of them no matter how different they may be in other parts of their doctrine, are going to encourage their followers to do some kind of fasting along the way. This is because they know the power of working with fasting, how it can clean out the spirit and the body and can provide a whole bunch of other benefits in the process as well. It is interesting to see how these thoughts have moved from different parts of the world, and even from philosophy to religion and it is seen as a good thing for the body.

Another group that is going to focus on fasting is going to be those who partake in yogic practices. These are going to date back thousands of years. Paramahansa Yogananda says, "Fasting is a natural method of healing". And to this day, those who work with what is known as Ayurveda, or ancient healing practice, will include some form of fasting as a therapy.

Fasting in the modern world

It is true that fasting has been seen as an important thing when it comes to the past, and with many of the major religions and thinkers of our world. But where does fasting seem to fit in when we talk about the modern world? Today, we often see that healers and different physicians who work with more of a spiritual or holistic orientation with their patients are going to recommend fasting on a regular basis to help improve health. This is because our conventional Western medicine is not going to fully embrace this natural remedy all of the ways. But, we are seeing that this kind of medicine is starting to accept more of the body to mind connection, and as this grows, it is likely that more doctors and practitioners are going to be willing to work with ideas like fasting to help with healing.

There is also more and more scientific research that proves there is an unseen energy that is directed through the body that is able to naturally incline the body to be healthy and balanced if we allow it. Even Dr. Mehmet Oz, M.D. has said that he believes that the future or our medical world is going to lie in studying the patterns of energy that go through the body, and that we need to learn how to enhance these patterns in a more positive manner to get better health results.

The idea here is that if a body is not directed towards healing spiritually, emotionally, or physically, then no medical procedure or amount of surgery is going to be able to change this. Any scientist is going to concede that only the body itself is going to be able to take the tissues and restore them and restore them back to their original state of perfection.

While there are a lot of great medical advances out there, there are also times when medication and other cures are pushed because they cost a lot of money, or because they are able to quickly mask the problem, rather than actually helping out with it. You may feel better, but the underlying cause is still going to be there, and that is a problem.

But when we choose to work with remedies that are more natural, we find that these will succeed in gearing the other aspects, such as the mental emotional, and spiritual parts of our being, towards wanting to be healthy. Fasting is one of these natural methods that we are able to use to help benefit us and give us the results that we want.

It is amazing what fasting is able to do for us. It has been used for many thousands of years to help heal and for many other emotional and spiritual things. Even a short fast that only lasts for one day is able to bring about a lot of big and small changes to our overall psyche, which can make it a great option to add in, no matter what kind of health condition you are fighting, or even which one you are trying to prevent.

Chapter 4: Myths about Intermittent Fasting

Because of an increasing amount of misunderstanding when it comes to intermittent fasting, it is likely that you have heard some kind of myth about this fasting and you think that it is a bad thing to do. You may assume that fasting is going to cause you more harm than good. You may assume that you are going to gain weight when you go on it. And you may assume that it is going to be really bad for your metabolism and you won't be able to fix the mistake if it goes wrong.

There are a number of myths and misunderstandings that come with intermittent fasting, and getting these out of the way will make it easier to understand how this kind of diet plan is going to work, and why it may be the best option for you to work with!

If you miss breakfast, you are going to gain weight.

One of the myths that we have heard for many years is that breakfast is considered the most important meal of the day. There is a myth that breakfast is going to be super special and it is a meal that you just should never miss. Although there are some observational studies out there that show that skipping breakfast can be linked to obesity and being overweight this is going to be more about the person, rather than the fact that you miss breakfast.

The idea here is that the people who miss breakfast are often going to overcompensate. They won't eat what they need in order to keep themselves happy and full of good nutrients. They are going to eat as much as possible for lunch and overdo it, and this causes them to gain more weight when they skip.

The thing that is interesting here is that the matter of whether breakfast is the most important meal of the day, or if it is better for you to skip it. This study was published in 2014, and it was done in order to compare whether eating breakfast or skipping breakfast was better in 283 obese or overweight adults. After the study went on for 16 weeks, it shows that there wasn't a difference in weight between the two.

What this shows us is that there isn't going to be much of a difference with your weight loss or gain based on whether you eat breakfast or not. So, just because you go on the intermittent fast and you are missing out on your first meal of the day or putting it back by a few hours, you are not going to gain a lot of weight in the process.

If breakfast is a pain for you to get to because you are so busy or you find that your intermittent fasting schedule works out the best for you if you are able to miss out on breakfast rather than one of the other meals, then go for it. Just because you missed breakfast does not mean that you are going to end up gaining weight when you are on a fast, as long as your other habits are as healthy as possible in the process.

Eating on a regular basis is going to boost your metabolism

There is a big myth out there that you need to eat five or six times a day in order to keep your metabolism burning. The idea here is that smaller meals many times a day are going to make it so that your metabolism will keep going strong and will burn through more calories. While it is true that your body is going to speed up and use some more energy to burn through food, research suggests that it really doesn't matter how many meals you eat, it matters how many calories. If you eat 2000 calories, it doesn't matter if you spread it between two meals or six meals, your body is going to expend the same number of calories.

Eating more often is going to fight off the hunger

There are a lot of people who assume that when you eat a lot of meals or your snack often, you are going to be able to fight off cravings and any excessive hunger. There have been a few different studies that talk about this, but you will find that the results are mixed. Some studies are going to suggest that eating more often is going to reduce hunger, and other studies find that this isn't going to have any effects. And then some studies show that this is actually going to increase the levels of hunger you have.

Basically, it is going to be more likely that this is based on the individual. If you find that snacking is best for you and can make it so that you experience fewer cravings overall, and prevent you from binging, then this may be better for you. But since there isn't a lot of evidence that eating more or snacking is going to reduce your hunger, and you will find that working with intermittent fasting can be a better option for you.

In fact, for most people eating more often is going to cause more problems overall. They find that each time they bring out a snack or eat another meal introduces them to more temptation to eat more food and calories than they need. When they are able to limit themselves to just a few meals a day, it ends up allowing them to eat meals that are larger, while still maintaining their calorie counts for the day.

The brain has to have glucose to keep up

There are some people who think that if you are not consuming carbs every few hours, then the brain is going to struggle with doing well. This is based on the idea that our brains are only able to use glucose in order to stay fueled up and ready to go. However, what we forget to bring into the discussion is that the body is able to produce the glucose that it needs through a process that is known as gluconeogenesis. This is usually something that is not needed but the liver is able to use the stored glycogen to help supply the brain for many hours. There will be plenty of fuel to get you through a short fast.

When you fast, you put your body into starvation mode

One of the arguments that are out there when it comes to intermittent fasting is that it is going to end up putting your body into what is known as starvation mode. According to some of the claims, not eating is going to make your body feel like it is starving, and once that happens, the body will shut down your metabolism and will make it hard to burn fat.

It is true that long-term weight loss is going to end up reducing the number of calories that you end up burning. This is the starvation mode, but that is more because your body is going to need less energy to get around because you are carrying around less weight over time. This has nothing to do with the fast at all.

In fact, there have been studies done that show how fasting for a time frame up to 48 hours is actually going to be able to boost your metabolism up to 14 percent. You do not want to go on a fast that is much longer than that though. Fasts that are longer than the 48 hours can end up reversing the effect and will force the metabolism to go down compared to the baseline, causing it to burn fewer calories to reserve energy.

Another study that was done on this topic showed that fasting on alternate days for a time period of 22 days did not lead the metabolism to decrease, but the participants were able to lose 4 percent of their fat mass, an impressive feat for those who were dealing with a fast for three weeks.

The good news is that intermittent fasting, in all of the protocols, is not going to ask you to go for more than 24 hours of fasting at a time. This is perfect because it keeps you under the 48-hour limit, and will help you to increase your metabolism, even if you are not eating as often.

Fasting is bad because it makes you lose muscles

Another myth that we need to watch out for is the idea that intermittent fasting is going to make you lose out on your muscle tone. It is true that this can happen when you go on a diet in general, but there is no evidence that it is going to happen more with fasting than it does with any other dieting method. There are even some studies that will show us how fasting could make it easier to maintain more of your muscle mass while you are losing weight.

In one review study that was completed, intermittent calorie restriction is going to cause a similar amount of weight loss as we can see with restricting calories, but the reduction in your muscle mass is going to be less. In another study, participants were supposed to eat the same amount of calories that they usually did, but these calories were supposed to be saved for one big meal in the night, rather than spread throughout the day. The people in this study ended up losing body fat while also having a modest increase in their muscle mass.

As you can see, intermittent fasting is not going to make the muscles fade away. At best, it could be the link that you are looking for when you want to be able to gain some more muscle and maintain it while losing weight. In the worst case, it isn't going to make you lose any more muscle mass than what you would see with any other weight loss plan.

Intermittent fasting is going to make you eat too much

There are a lot of people who worry about going on a fast because they feel that they won't be able to lose weight due to them eating too much when it is time to eat again.

This is something that could be partly true. After a fast, people are going to often eat a bit more than if they hadn't been fasting. This means that they are more likely to compensate for the calories that they lose during that fasting period because they will eat more during the following meals. However, as long as you don't pig out and go crazy, the compensation is not going to be complete.

There was one study that showed that people who fasted for the whole day only ended up eating an additional 500 calories on the following day. So, they would expend about 2400 calories during the fasting day, then they would overeat by 500 calories on their eating day. The total calorie reduction that would be seen here is 1900 calories, which is actually a large amount to give up in just two days!

The neat thing about intermittent fasting is that it is going to be able to naturally reduce the amount of food that you take in while also boosting your metabolism. It is going to reduce your insulin levels, boost the human growth hormone, and can increase your norepinephrine levels as well.

Because of all these factors and more, intermittent fasting is going to make it easier to lose weight and fat rather than gain it. And this is exactly what a lot of people are looking for when they want to improve their health. You have to be a bit careful about what you are eating and make sure that you monitor it a little bit overall, but you will find that if you are able to stick with it, and you don't go crazy with what you are eating the next day to make up for your fasts, that intermittent fasting is the best way to lose the weight that you want, rather than making you overeat and gain weight.

These are just a few of the different myths that you may hear about when you are dealing with intermittent fasting and what it is going to do for your overall health. Learning what is the truth and what is not can make a big difference in how much you rely on and trust this kind of diet plan. When you are ready to finally lose weight and feel you're very best while improving your mind and body, putting some of these myths to rest and learning as much about the intermittent fast is going to be super important to help you see results.

Chapter 5: What Happens to the Body During a Fast?

The next thing that we need to take some time to explore is what will happen to the body when it goes on a fast. There are some people who hear about this kind of eating plan and they worry about the idea of fasting. They may be heard about fasting in the past and they worry about the ways that this is going to work against them, and how fasting is just going to slow down their metabolism, make them feel sick, and will just work against any of their weight loss goals in the process.

The reality of the matter is that fasting can actually be healthy for you, as long as you don't overdo it and go crazy. If you plan to fast for a month or you fast with just a few hundred calories a day all of the time, then yes this is going to backfire and make you sick. But intermittent fasting makes sure that you do not fast for too long at a given time, and all of the protocols for intermittent fasting that we will talk about later are completely safe to work with.

With this in mind, we need to take a quick look at fasting and what all it is going to entail. When you go on a fast, the body is going to find that the constant stream of food that you provided in the past is now gone, at least for a bit. Instead, the body has to figure out the way that it will be able to generate some of its own energy, rather than relying on you to supply this.

Think of it this way, when a device is plugged in, it is able to take energy right from the socket and from the wall. When you unplug it, the device has to rely on the batter it has. This is what is going to happen when you work with intermittent fasting. You are pulling the plug on the body temporarily and asking it to rely on its own personal batter in order to give you the energy that you need.

You will find during this that the liver is actually going to be one of the biggest players when we work with this process. This is because the liver can come into play and start taking the stored fat found in the body and then convert those into ketone bodies. These ketone bodies are going to the things that you will rely on during the fast to give you the energy that you need.

This is very similar to what you see with the ketogenic diet. Even if you do not go on a diet plan that is similar to the keto diet, fasting will react in the same way. When you do not have a constant source of carbs coming into your body, which happens when you are not eating for a prolonged period of time, the body will switch over to the fact that you have stored up. Fat is a very efficient energy source, which results in you not only burning up all that belly fat that has been holding onto your body, you will also have more energy in the process. If you add fasting to the ketogenic diet, and the fat burning process will get so much better.

There are a lot of great benefits that come with fasting, but detoxification is one of the biggest. Detoxification is actually a regular process in the body and it will occur when the skin, lymph glands, lungs, kidney, liver, and colon neutralize or eliminate toxins that build up in the body. When you go on an intermittent fast, this process will speed up because the body works to break down fats. Toxins and chemicals that you get from the environment and from food, and which are stored in the body in your fat reserves, will naturally be released when you go on a fast.

Putting your body through detox is going to be so important to your good health. Thanks to the foods that we eat or poor diets, and just the toxins, stress, and more from our lifestyles and the world around us, a lot of gunk and bad stuff is going to get stuck in the body. In fact, just the idea that the body is repairing and working on adding new parts all of the time and removing old parts tells us that a lot of stuff can get stuck in the body.

Unless we go through a good detox, which is really effective when we decide to go on a fast, we are going to leave all of those dead and old parts, all of the damage, and all of the toxins floating around in the body. And this is never going to spell anything that is good for us. It basically means that we have a lot of work to do if we are looking to get our bodies in better health. In fact, the more of this bad stuff that is found in the body, and the longer it is allowed to stick around and accumulate, the worse it is going to be for our health.

And this is where a fast is going to come in handy a lot of the time. You will find that when you go on a fast, you are giving the body some time to empty itself of all of these bad things in no time at all. It is more effective than any of the other detoxes that you may have used in the past, and it is going to rely on some of the natural processes of the body in order to get it done. How cool is that!

In addition to detoxing all those bad chemicals that are in the body, fasting is good for so many other reasons. It is a great tool to heal the body and mine. Looking at the physical level, resources and energy are taken away from the digestive system (which is always in use if you are someone who grazes on food all day long) and that energy is moved over to other processes in the body. This can include processes that allow the body to better heal, rebuild, and replenish itself. This is why those who go on an intermittent fast often have more energy, fewer health conditions, and are even better able to lose weight and body fat compared to others.

There are always times when we need to allow the body to heal itself. We could take a bunch of medicine to make this happen, and sometimes this is what we end up having to do to help the body along. But sometimes the body is going to do its best work when it is allowed to do the work on its own. If we don't give it a chance to do this by taking care of it, then this is something that is never going to happen.

With this in mind, fasting is going to allow us to make this happen. Often the reason that we are not healing or that we are dealing with a negative disease is that the body is not allowed to cleanse itself. Since we are stuck in the first phase of our bodybuilding and trying to repair things, but we do not allow the damaged and old stuff to be removed, these old and damaged parts just stick around.

They get in the way, and they don't allow the body to come in and heal anything because they are in the way. Since fasting allows for this to happen, it is going to be a lifesaver in terms of healing. You will naturally give your body a chance to come in and clear out some of the old and damaged things, which can sometimes be all that you need to heal the body. And if not, simply by removing those parts and giving the wounded parts some room to breathe is going to be enough to help you to start the healing process that you need.

The neat thing about this is that there have actually been studies done over the years that shows us how during a fast, there is going to be signs that abnormal growth in tissue, such as what we see with tumors and cancer, are going to be starved of the nutrients that they need during this time. When this happens it is easier for the body to break them down and they can be removed as you detox your body during the fast.

In addition, you will find that going on a regular fast like this is going to help you have healthier organs, tissues, and cells. This is going to happen due to the fact that fasting is going to make it easier for the body to tap into the resources that it already has. The body will then refocus all of its energy on building down at the microscopic levels. This means that it is going to look at the genes of DNA and RNA, ensuring that the cells and the tissues of the body are built in the right manner each time.

Now, it is likely that you have heard rumors in the past that going on a fast is going to end up slowing down the metabolism and making it harder for you to maintain or lose weight in the process. This is why so many people are scared to even skip a meal ever. But think of it this way. If you have ever been sick, you may have missed eating a few meals, and it is possible that you even skipped eating for a few days while you dealt with the bug.

Do you think it is likely that missing those few meals during recovery was really that big of a deal and that you are doomed forever? In reality, those fasts probably helped you to get better faster because you allowed the body to use the energy it would have needed to digest your food to go and fight off the infection. While you may have only been thinking about those facts in terms of how sick you were and how you were not able to keep anything down, it was actually a time when the body was probably working extra hard to heal itself, and you were doing something that was so wonderful for the body.

This is kind of the same idea. If you do the protocols of fasting the right way and make sure that you are taking in enough calories to make the body happy with lots of nutrients, then you are not going to have to worry about intermittent fasting slowing down your metabolism at all. In fact, you are going to realize, just like many others who have gone on an intermittent fast in the past, that when you follow the protocol in the right manner, you can actually help to speed up your metabolism in the process, making weight loss much easier overall.

While there are going to be a ton of misconceptions when it comes to working with fasting, you will find that it is actually one of the best things that you are able to do with your body. It is going to help you to clear out the body and can change up the way that the body is going to work as a result as well. Even after just a few short fasts, you are going to find that the body is more energized, that it feels better overall, and that you are going to be able to notice a big difference in how well you heal while a reduction in the cases of bad health diseases goes to a minimum as well.

Chapter 6: Different Fasting Techniques

One of the neat things about going on a fast is that you can actually choose from a few different techniques that you want to use before starting. There isn't a one size fits all here, which is one of the things that makes the intermittent fast something that is so wonderful to work with for everyone. If you don't think that you can make it all day long without eating, there are fasting methods that work for that. If you are worried about snacking if you start eating, or not being able to stop, then you can find some methods that work well for that.

As you have been going through this guidebook, you may have worried a bit about the different fasting techniques and whether they would be too hard for you to follow or not. But you will find that while some of they may be a bit easier to follow, especially in the beginning when you are not used to doing fasting at all, that they are still going to help you to lose weight and improve your overall health. Some may provide the results a little bit faster, but all of them are going to work.

With that in mind, let's take a look at some of the different types of intermittent fasting that you are able to choose:

Leangains or 16/8 fasting

Most people who go on intermittent fasting will choose to go with the 16/8 method. With this method, you are required to fast for 14 to 16 hours each day, and then the remainder of the day you are technically able to eat whatever you would like. With this eating window, you still have enough time to eat two or three meals without too many issues, so it is still easy to fit this eating schedule into your day without feeling restricted.

This is a really easy method to follow, especially if you pick the right hours to do your fasting. For example, simply stop eating supper around seven or eight at night and do not have any late night snacks. When you get to the next day, you will skip breakfast and start eating around noon. This will put you into a 16 hour fast. If you like to eat breakfast, just stop eating around five at night and have breakfast at nine in the morning. You must be careful to not take any late night snacks in while you are on this plan, but it is much easier compared to some of the other options you may choose.

The biggest issue that comes with this option is that some people feel hungry when they wake up in the morning or they have breakfast as part of their morning routine. You can still have breakfast, you just need to move it a little bit later in the morning rather than eating it the moment you get up. For example, you could have breakfast at nine or ten in the morning, you just need to stop eating supper a little bit earlier.

Studies have shown that both men and women are able to benefit from this method of intermittent fasting. However, it is usually best to go with a little shorter fasting period. Women respond well to the daily fast, but they see the best results when they make their fasting window be between 14 to 15 hours instead of going as long.

During your fasting window, you are able to have coffee, water, and other non-caloric beverages so that you are not dehydrated. Drinking plenty of water can also be the answer you need to prevent some of those hunger pains. When it comes to eating, you should stick with foods that are healthy. You are technically allowed to eat anything that you want with your fasting, but eating a bunch of junk is not going to help you with your health goals. Sticking with a good diet plan, or at least eating healthier foods, will make intermittent fasting more effective.

You are allowed to pick out the eating and fasting windows that work for you as long as the fasting window is a bit longer. Some people stick with fasting for sixteen hours, while others will go with eighteen hours, twenty hours, or even fourteen hours. Pick the time that helps you to stick on the fast better and that works the best for your daily routine.

Another option with the 5:2 diet

Another method that you are able to work with when it comes to intermittent fasting is known as the 5:2 diet. This one is going to have you eat in a normal manner (though you should try to eat foods that are as healthy as possible on those days), and then on the other two days, your calories are going to be restricted. During your fasting days, you need to stick with 500 calories for women and 600 calories for men for the whole day.

When picking out your fasting days, make sure that they are not consecutive. You want to spread them out through the week. Other than not having them be right next to each other, you are able to pick any day of the week to make into your fasting one.

When you are fasting, you get to choose whether you would like to have all of your calories in one bigger meal at the end of the day, or if you would like to split them up and have the meals throughout the day. Try to go with foods that are full of nutrients and will do your body good rather than filling up and wasting your calories on a donut or something similar. And on your non-fasting days, make sure that you are picking out meals that have a lot of nutrition as well to help you stay healthy and not starve yourself.

Eat stop eat

Now we are going to work with the eat stop eat method of fasting. This one is going to be a bit more difficult compared to the others because there are going to be more days when you need to fast but it is going to be one that gives you some good results and will help you to really cut out the carvings that you are feeling and more.

When you decide to use the eat stop eat plan, your goal is to go on a fast that lasts 24 hours two times a week. You can pick the days that work the best for you with this one, just make sure that you are not going two days in a row. Maybe you will pick the two days that you are going to be the busiest for the week anyway. Then you don't have to worry about finding time to eat or making meals during that time. You can spend that time working on getting things done and being more productive, and then eat later.

It's not as difficult as it sounds. You can choose to stop eating after supper one day and then not eat until supper the next day. You are never going longer than that and can choose to go from one lunch to the next or from one breakfast to the next. Most people like to go with the first choice, going from supper to supper because it allows them to never go to bed hungry with this plan.

Trying alternate day fasting

This type of fasting can be one of the hardest to follow because it requires the most days that you will need to fast throughout the week. But if you work it outright, it can make your week easier because you will not need to plan as many meals as out as you normally would.

With the alternate day fasting option, you will fast every other day. You can choose whether those fasting days will allow you to 500 calories or less during the day or if you will completely fast and not have anything to eat during your fasting day. This is seen as the most effective method of fasting because most of the studies done on intermittent fasting that show how well it works to focus on alternate day fasting.

The idea of alternate day fasting may be effective, but it is one of the most difficult ones to go with. You will need to go into a fast every other day, which is a lot harder than what you would do with some of the other fasting options. You may decide to build up to this a little bit, starting with two days a week of fasting and then moving to three a week until you end up fasting every other day for the best results.

If you have gotten started with alternate day fasting and find that it is too hard for you to follow, then it is fine to try out something else. This is one of the more difficult options to go with and it is not for everyone. If you need to add a few calories into the day to make it easier, to change over to a different method of fasting, that is fine. All of them are effective and can help you to lose weight, you just need to find the method that works the best for you.

Warrior diet

The next option that we are going to look at, and the final one, for now, is known as the Warrior Diet. This is a popular diet plan, but it is going to prove to be a bit difficult. The goal with this one is too fast for 20 hours each day and then fit your meals into just four hours during the day. This can be restrictive, and it may be best to start with one of the other methods, such as the 16/8 method and then build up for this.

There are some options here to eat small amounts of fruits and vegetables during the fast. But often this needs to be kept to fewer than 200 calories of those a day, and it could be difficult to restrict yourself rather than overeating with it. But for the most part, you will need to save your calories for that four-hour window.

In addition, this option of intermittent fasting is going to have a meal plan attached. While others encourage you to eat wholesome and nutrient-rich foods, the Warrior diet asks followers to go with a diet that is similar to the Paleo diet. This helps to make it even more effective for those who are looking to lose weight and improve their health.

The Warrior Diet

Another option that you can choose to go with is known as the Warrior Diet. This one is going to be similar to what we saw when we took a look at the 16/8 plan, but the fasting window is going to be a bit longer. This one is going to ask you to reduce your eating window down to just four hours a day. This means that over the course of the day, you are going too fast for 20 hours, and then you can eat what you would like for the rest of the day.

As you can imagine, this is going to be a good way to restrict the number of calories that you are able to eat during the day. Unless you decide to eat a pound of cheesecake and lots of other bad foods during this time, you will find that it is hard for you to overeat when you go on this kind of diet plan. Instead, you are going to eat fewer calories, while giving your body lots of time to really rev up the metabolism so that you can lose a bit more along the way.

There are some versions of the Warrior Diet that are going to allow you to eat a few calories during the day. You can graze a bit on some fruits and vegetables if you would like. But this needs to stick to as low as possible. If you have trouble stopping yourself from eating when you start, then it is best if you are able to just stay away from this and save all of you're eating for that four-hour eating window later on.

Many people who go on the Warrior diet are going to also follow the Paleo diet. This is an all-natural diet plan that asks you to basically eat foods that are similar to what you are able to find in nature if you were a hunter or a gatherer. This includes lots of fish, berries, some vegetables, and even meats. You do not need to go on this kind of diet plan if you feel that it is going to be too hard, and as long as you eat foods that are wholesome and nutritious, you are going to be just fine.

Many people who want to do bodybuilding and other similar strength training adventures are going to like going on the Warrior diet. This one is easy to maintain and will help you to really lean out and get rid of the body fat. However, if you had a really unhealthy eating plan or diet in the past, starting out with this tough one right from the beginning is going to be hard. If this is your goal, you may want to consider starting out with the 16/8 diet plan and then building up to this.

Skipping meals randomly

This is one that you can try out if you just want to prepare your body for intermittent fasting or if you just don't want to spend all that much time worrying about when you are able to eat in order to lose the weight. With this one, you do not need to worry so much about following one of the more structured intermittent fasting plans to get the benefits. With it, you will just skip some meals from time to time. These can be when you are not hungry or when you are just too busy to have a meal. It is a big myth that you have to eat something every few hours in order to avoid starvation mode or you will start to lose out on muscle tone.

The body is well adapted to handle longer time periods without needing to eat. It is not like our ancestors were not always able to get the food that they wanted or needed and they were just fine. Missing out on a few meals, especially if you are not all that hungry or too busy, is not going to be that big of a deal.

Any time that you end up skipping a meal or two, you are technically going to be on this kind of fast. If you are too busy to grab a breakfast on the way out the door, just make sure that you eat a healthy lunch and dinner. If you are on the run and you just are not able to find someplace to eat, then it is fine to miss out on a meal. This is not going to cause you any harm and will actually help you to save time and not have to worry about all the planning that can happen with intermittent fasting with some of the other methods.

This one is nice to work with because you will not have to worry so much about it as you will with some of the others. This one you just miss a meal here and there when it works for you. You probably won't see as good of results with this one compared to some of the others because you are not getting all the regularity of fasting that you do with them, but it is better than nothing and is a lot easier to work with. Perhaps try to skip a meal or two during the week if you are really trying to get some good results with your weight loss, but otherwise, you can just miss some meals when it works for you.

There are a lot of different options that you can make when it comes to fasting. And all of the methods are going to provide you with results and a ton of benefits. Now the choice is to figure out which one is going to fit the best into your lifestyle and will help you to reach your goals.

Chapter 7: What Comes with Fasting

The neat thing about working with intermittent fasting is that it allows you to work on a lot of different types of health concerns that you have. It is one of the healthiest ways to take care of yourself and your body while preventing a lot of the disorders and diseases that we talked about earlier in this guidebook. With this in mind, it is important to take some time to explore fasting and what it can mean to your health, and some of the reasons that you may want to give it a try.

Healthy brain function

If you are looking to get a healthier brain, then you need to take a look at intermittent fasting. New research has indicated that fasting is able to really help the brain, and this includes the fact that it is able to even help reduce how aging is going to change up the brain. It has been known for a long time that bouts of intermittent fasting are able to provide us with relief from inflammation throughout the whole body. And now leading scientists think that fasting is going to be able to improve the health of your brain and could be one of the biggest things you can do to maximize the functioning of the brain.

Researchers at the National Institute of Aging in Baltimore have spent some time reviewing the literature and have also performed studies to help us see the positive effects of fasting on the brain and how this helps keep the brain smart. According to Professor Mark Mattson, the head of the laboratory of NeuroSciences for this study, these benefits don't come just from the calorie restriction, but mostly from the intentional periods of fasting.

The first benefit that we are going to see comes from the building and cleansing phases of the body. When we eat, it is going to stimulate the body to go into a building phase so that it is able to store both toxins and nutrients that we take in. this is an essential phase because it helps us to build up new tissues and cells, and ensures that we store up nutrients for times when food and nutrients are not as plentiful. We will see that this phase is going to be led mostly through the insulin hormone.

When we begin to go on a fast that is longer than 6 hours, we are going to enter into what is known as the cleansing phase. This is going to be a phase where the body tears down cells that are old and damaged. This is going to turn on what is known as brain autophagy, or self-eating. This may sound bad, but it is basically where the cells are going to recycle waste material, repair themselves, and more. These repair processes are going to happen when the human growth hormone is released.

Because fasting allows us to have some time to work on the cleansing process in the body, it is going to be one of the most powerful methods that we can use in order to boost immunity, enhance how well the tissues can heal, and even reduce inflammation. This is easy to do simply by going a few hours without eating.

The next thing to look at here is the idea that fasting is going to boost the human growth hormone. This hormone is able to create what is known as a physiological change in our metabolism, one that is going to favor protein sparing and fat burning. The amino acids and proteins are going to be utilized in order to improve the neuron processing that goes on in the brain. They will also take the time to repair the collagen in the tissues, which is going to be a great thing when you want to improve the functionality and the strength that comes with your bones, ligaments, tendons, and muscles.

Researchers at the Intermountain Medical Center Heart Institute looked at how fasting was going to influence the levels of HGH in individuals. Men who had gone on a fast for 24 hours found that they had an increase of 2000 percent for circulating HGH. Women who were tested saw that their HGH levels increased by 1300 percent. This is huge especially when combined with the fact that these participants also say that their blood sugars stabilized, and their cholesterol levels improved while on a fast.

When all of this comes together, and the body is allowed to actually go through a process of cleaning itself out rather than just building up more things and adding in more toxins, it is going to get healthier overall. And this is exactly what fasting allows us to do.

Not only are the various organs of the body going to get a chance to clean themselves out, so will the brain. When the brain is not constantly hit by insulin and all of the reactions that come with that, and it is allowed to go through and clean out the toxins that have been sitting around, you are going to see a lot of benefits in the process. You will notice that you are able to think better, that there is less stress, that your brain fog is gone, and even some of your risk of developing dementia and Alzheimer's will fade away.

Weight loss

There are a lot of different ways that intermittent fasting is able to help you to improve your health and even lose weight. Many of the benefits that we have been talking about in this guidebook can come to mind, and just the fact that you are reducing the amount of time you get to eat during the day effectively cutting down calories because you are not allowed to snack and graze all of the time, can make a difference as well.

The main reason that you are going to see some weight loss when you decide to go on an intermittent fast is that this method of eating is going to make it easier to eat fewer calories on a regular basis. No matter which protocol you decide to go on, you will be going through a period of fasting, where you will skip one or more meals. Unless you go really crazy and eat at a buffet to make up for it each time, this is going to result in a calorie deficit overall. This is exactly what you need to see some weight loss. A

According to a study that was done in 2014 intermittent fasting can be a good way for you to lose a significant amount of weight in a short amount of time. With this particular study, intermittent fasting was found to reduce the weight of those following it by 3 to 8 percent over a period of 3 to 24 weeks depending on how long they were in the study and how long they did the fasting. These individuals were able to lose about .55 pounds per week with intermittent fasting by 1.65 pounds a week when they did alternate day fasting. In addition, they saw somewhere between 4 to 7 percent reduction in their waist circumference while on this plan as well.

This is a significant amount of weight for anyone to lose in such a short time, in six months or less, it is possible to lose up to eight percent of your body weight! And it can all be done without feeling like you are depriving yourself or being hungry all of the time and it isn't even that hard to follow!

Although it is not usually a requirement to count calories when you are on an intermittent fast, you are still going to need to moderate the number of calories that you are consuming in order to get the best results. It is not going to help you out much if you take in 3000 calories a day with limited amounts of movement, even if you are following one of the intermittent fasting protocols.

If you are able to make sure that your calories are limited at least a bit, and you can try to monitor what you take in on a daily basis, you will find that it is easier to lose weight. This can make it easier to stick with the plan without feeling like you are deprived all of the time, and it ensures that you are not going to be snacking all day long, or being tempted by some of those higher calorie foods and treats all of the time.

For those who struggle with losing weight because they graze all of the time or those who worry about overeating, intermittent fasting could be the way to control that a little bit. It will allow you a chance to get your snacking under control because you are only allowed to eat during certain times of the day. While over the long term you will lose similar amounts of weight with intermittent fasting as you will with calorie restriction on its own, usually calorie restriction is harder to do on its own, and you have to cut out the calories much more than you do with the fasts.

Because of this, many people prefer to go on a fast when it is time for them to lose weight. It allows them to restrict their calories in a more natural manner, and sometimes the mentality that you are not allowed to eat during the day or during a certain time is going to be more effective at keeping you on track compared to some other choices. Altogether, this comes and helps you to restrict your calories, increase your metabolism, and ensure that you are going to get the best results in the process with your weight loss goals.

Intermittent fasting can protect the brain

If you are looking for a way to protect the brain, then intermittent fasting is the option that you want to go with. There was one animal study that showed how intermittent fasting is able to enhance how well your brain functions and it can even help to protect against changes in your memory and learning function when compared against a control group.

This will help you in several ways. To start, intermittent fasting can help you out with creative and critical thinking, remembering important dates, and keeping your memories safe. This can help you to avoid so much brain fog and will make you feel better in no time.

In addition, there have been some studies that show how intermittent fasting is able to help prevent against some degenerative diseases. Going on one of these fasts and maintaining a healthy lifestyle may be the key to preventing Parkinson's and Alzheimer's disease.

Can boost your energy levels

For those who feel sluggish part way through the day, and feel like it is time for a nap by lunch time, low energy levels are a big problem. You may spend a lot of time drinking coffee, soda, and energy drinks in an attempt to help you feel better and to increase your levels of energy. But even though these may give you a little jolt and help you keep going, they are not going to be as positive as working with the root of the problem, and solving what is actually causing the problem.

Even though food is meant to give us energy, our poor diets and lifestyle are making us feel sick and tired all of the time. We eat more and take in more food and other substances in the hopes of giving us more energy overall, but this is just temporary, and it is going to just make you feel more worn out at the end of the day.

Intermittent fasting is going to be able to provide you with the energy that you are looking for. It is able to help you increase your energy in several ways, and they are all natural and great for you!

The first way that intermittent fasting is going to help you with your levels of energy is that it helps you to eat foods that are healthier and more wholesome for you. When you eat fruits and vegetables, and lots of good whole grains and protein sources, you will find that all of the great nutrition that is found inside these can give you energy that lasts for days.

Just by eating foods that are healthier, which is highly encouraged on this kind of eating plan, you will be able to see more energy. It will be easier to get up in the morning, you won't need that pick up in the middle of the day, and you can go into the evening with enough energy to get what you would like done rather than wanting to go to bed!

In addition to eating healthier foods that provide you with energy, the way that the intermittent fasting works will provide you with more energy as well. You will spend a bit of your time each week without providing the body with a new source of fuel. With traditional diets in America, you rely on lots of carbs for your fuel. This isn't necessarily a bad thing and you don't need to completely cut the carbs out. But these carbs are going to make it more difficult to control yourself because they are not efficient.

Often, even when you take in a lot of carbs already, the body is not going to be able to deal with them very efficiently. They will give you some energy, but way too soon the energy is gone. This forces us to either feel tired, or take in more of the carbs to help us to feel better and get more energy. It never seems like enough and then we end up in a cycle that just goes on and on and makes us unhealthy, and still low on energy.

When you go on a fast that keeps you away from the carbs for a bit, and you limit how many carbs that you eat during the eating times the body has to search for another source of energy. It isn't like the body turns off during this time. It still needs to function and move. The source that the body goes to is the fat reserves, and this can be great news for your energy levels!

The body may not be used to turning to the fat reserves to help you get energy for daily activities, but it is a really efficient source of fuel. You will find that may allowing the body to rely on these reserves, you are able to see a big jump in your energy levels, even when you cut down on the amount of time that you are allowed to eat each day.

Kicks the brain fog away

Do you deal with a lot of brain fog? Are you constantly dealing with problems remembering where you left things, important dates, or why you entered a room. Is it easy for you to make a lot of mistakes during the day because your mind just feels like it is in a fog all of the time?

Brain fog is something that a lot of people are dealing with on a regular basis, but they are not certain how they are going to be able to fix it. They may try to take a nap or do something healthy, but in reality, it is likely that they will take in some caffeine or another stimulant and hope that is enough to help them feel better and get things done.

With this said, intermittent fasting is going to be one of the best ways that you can kick away that brain fog and improve your concentration and your memory. Thanks to the healthy foods, the weight loss, and the timing of your meals, your brain is going to feel clearer and more ready to take on the day.

Often brain fog is going to be caused by the continuous supply of carbs and sugars that you provide to the brain and to the body. You may crave these, but the work that it takes to deal with them and use them up properly, can be exhausting to you. And often the excess is going to be enough to make the brain tired and add in some of the brain fog that you are used to feeling.

When you go through intermittent fasting, you get to deal with this problem. This doesn't mean that you have to give up carbs, but you do give the brain a break from how many carbs you take in. And because your eating window is so much smaller, it is less likely that you will overeat on these carbs, helping the brain to clear out, and think more critically in the long run.

Helps you to sleep better

Another benefit that you will be able to enjoy when you decide to go on an intermittent fasting is that it helps you to get more sleep in your life. Sleep is so important to our overall health, but many Americans are not getting the sleep that they need to feel their best. Many times we put sleep on hold. We have too many activities that we have to get done, from work to school to activities, to spending time with family, and more.

It is natural in our modern world to feel like we just don't have enough time to get everything done. And sleep is often the first thing to go. We feel that if we cut down on a few hours of sleep, that opens us up for doing more. The reality is, we really need to add back some sleep into our schedules, and cut out some of the other things.

What makes the problem worse is that not only do we not get enough hours of sleep at night, we often suffer from light sleep or restless sleep. This may be slightly better than no sleep at all, but it leaves us feeling groggy and irritated in the morning. Intermittent fasting is able to jump right in and help with all of this, giving us a deeper sleep when we get to bed, and encourages us to get enough hours of sleep in the day as well.

There are many conditions that can start to happen when you miss out on some of the sleep that your body needs. Your insulin resistance goes up, your blood pressure can go up from all the extra stress that you are carrying around due to lack of sleep, and you get irritated and angry more often. You may not feel like these things are bothering you, simply because you have been feeling this way for a very long time. But all of it comes together to make us miserable and ruins our health.

When you go on an intermittent fasting regimen, you find that some of these problems can be solved. You will get more sleep without insomnia or restless sleep at night, and wake up refreshed and ready to take on the day. Within just a few days of getting started on this diet plan, you will notice a difference in how well you sleep, how many aches and pains you have in the morning from bad sleep, in your mood, and even in your levels of energy.

For those who have already spend a lot of time dealing with sleep problems, and who may even be on sleep medications that don't seem to work, then an intermittent fast may be the right option to help you get some results. It is efficient, it helps you to improve your health, and what is better for your health than a good nights' sleep?

Can prevent the side effects of aging

There are people who follow the intermittent fasting because they believe that this is the way to keep themselves looking and feeling young. They believe that intermittent fasting will give them the tools to live a lot longer. There have not been many studies done on this simply because people have not been on intermittent fating to see if it is true.

All of us want to stay as young as possible. We have no want to look older than our age, and we would prefer it if we could look younger. But with a poor diet, weight gain, and other harmful stimulants that we seal with on a regular basis, it is no wonder that we start to look and feel older than our years.

This is where intermittent fasting is going to come into play. It is able to reverse some of the harm that we may have caused our bodies, and can make it easier to feel more energetic, to make the mind clearer, and even help get rid of acne, wrinkles, fine lines and more!

Helps you with your blood sugar levels

For those who are dealing with troubles when it comes to their blood sugar levels, intermittent fasting can be the option that you need to help deal with these higher levels, and get them under control to hopefully reduce your risk of diabetes, or make it easier to handle this disease if you are already dealing with it. Diabetes is becoming a big problem in our world, and learning how to cut it off and prevent it from happening can do some wonders for our health.

Due to the nature of intermittent fasting, and the different parts that come with it, you may find that your body reduces its resistance to insulin, and starts to feel better. When you stop the constant supply for carbs and sugars from sun up to sun down, you give the body time to fix itself and to heal anything that has been damaged. This is critical when it comes to stopping insulin resistance, and can make the body more receptive to the insulin and the glucose you do take in when it is time.

This doesn't mean that you have to completely give up carbs. Often just limiting your eating window during the week will be enough to help your body feel so much better. And many people choose to cut down their carbs, bringing them into a more reasonable level, to help you to feel better and to help the body heal from the damage that may have happened with your previous lifestyle. This will ensure that you are going to see some amazing benefits, and that you can prevent, and sometimes reverse, the effects of diabetes on your body.

Helps you to become more creative.

We have talked about some of the amazing brain benefits that can happen when you go on an intermittent fast, but we need to bring up one more here. If you have been struggling with problem solving, thinking critically, or coming up with solutions to problems that are more creative, then the intermittent fasting may be the right option for you.

When we aren't taking proper care of our bodies, we are going to find that there can be troubles when we try to think things through. We may forget things, have brain fog, and issues with thinking in a more critical manner. When we go on an intermittent fast and try to eat foods that are healthier for your body, you will be able to take better care of your body, and can help the mind to work better as well.

Imagine how it is going to feel when you can finally get rid of that brain fog, and when powerful and creative ideas start to come to you without as much struggle! You can remember where you left the car keys, you will remember what was said in an email a few weeks ago and make fewer mistakes at work, and you will be the one getting all of the great ideas to share with others, be better at problem solving, and can think critically when the need arises.

A healthier heart

All of us want to have a healthier heart. We look forward to a long life with few health conditions, and a big hope that we will actually be able to enjoy the retirement that we have with a healthy mind and heart. But with the traditional American diet, we end up failing here. There are a lot of things about the traditional American diet that are going to cause some stress on the heart, but going on an intermittent fast is going to help prevent some of these issues for us and will keep our heart going nice and strong.

When you can cut out some of the harmful foods, like the saturated fats, the sodium, and all of those carbs, sugars, and processed ingredients, you are doing the heart so much good. You are clearing out the plaque that has built up in the arteries, you are lowering the blood pressure, you are keeping the blood sugar levels in line, and hopefully you are reducing some of the stress that you feel as well. All of these come together to help you to make your heart as strong as possible.

Other neat things about intermittent fasting

We have just spent some time taking a look at two of the most well-known and common health benefits when we look at intermittent fasting. But the really neat thing here is that these are not the only benefits that you are going to be able to experience when you decide to go on a fast. Some of the other amazing health benefits that you may want to spend some time looking at, and which can be an added bonus to going on this kind of eating plan and improving your own life include:

- A decrease in your core body temperature. This happens because there is a little decline in general body functions and the metabolic rate of the individual.

- Blood sugar levels also start to drop. This is because the body will start to rely on the reserves of glycogen that have been stored in the liver rather than having to rely so much on the glucose and sugars you get in your diet.
- BMR, or base metabolic rate, is reduced to help conserve energy a bit.
- The digestive system, which you have overworked from all that eating, is given a chance to clean itself out and will be more efficient at nutrient absorption and digestion in the future.
- The lining in your intestines and your stomach will have time to restore the muscles and glands so that they can remove waste matter more efficiently.
- Hormone production starts to increase so that you can feel better.
- Anti-aging growth hormones kick in, helping you to look and feel younger.
- Weight loss. Many people go on intermittent fasting because it helps them to lose weight. With the digestive system being able to clear out and become more efficient, and your metabolism speeds up, you are able to burn more calories, and fat

than ever before, resulting in some amazing results.

Fasting can change a bunch of things in your body. Whether you go on a day fast a few times a week or you do some of the shorter fasts that are popular with intermittent fasting, you will be able to receive all the benefits above and more. Whether or not you choose to go with another diet plan in addition to this one or not, you will see some amazing results if you do intermittent fasting with a healthy lifestyle.

Chapter 8: How to Take the First Steps

Sometimes the hardest part about this diet plan is figuring out which steps you should take. You want to make sure that you are doing it the proper way, but you may be worried that it is going to be too hard or you are not going to do it the right way, which means a lot of hard work without being able to really see the results that you want.

This chapter is going to help you out with this. We are going to take a look at some of the first steps that you are able to use in order to really make sure that you are set and that you are able to see the benefits you want from intermittent fasting.

Recommendations on What to Eat

The first thing that we need to take a look at here is some of the foods that you should eat when you are going on an intermittent fast. Outside of the Warrior Diet, there isn't really a set diet plan that goes with any of the protocols for intermittent fasting. You could technically eat whatever you would like to through this method as long as you fit it into your eating window.

With that said, it is likely that you are not going to see weight loss or any health benefits if you fast and then only eat pizza, donuts, candy, pop, and other junk foods when you get to eat again. Having something as a splurge is just fine on occasion, but you will find that eating foods that are generally healthy for you are going to be the best option overall.

What this means is eating a diet that is full of healthy and wholesome foods, and eliminating the ones that are going to be seen as junk foods. There are a lot of people who choose to go on the ketogenic diet along with the intermittent fast because it helps them to burn through fat and see more weight loss in a short amount of time. You don't have to go on this diet plan though if it seems too hard or restrictive for you.

Focusing on a diet plan that has a lot of variety in it, and will ensure that your body is replenished with the nutrients it needs while fasting is what will be the most important. This means following a diet plan that includes a lot of healthy fruits and vegetables, healthy dairy products, lean protein, and whole grains can be critical. And adding in as much variety to these as possible so you are not eating the same foods each day can make it so much better too.

Adding in a little treat on occasion is not going to be such a big deal. And intermittent fasting is great because you don't have to rely on counting your calories as much. But you still want to remain mostly healthy in the foods that you are choosing while on this diet plan.

The trick when you are on this diet plan is that you need to make sure that the foods you consume are as healthy as possible. This is the only way to ensure that you are going to get the best benefits and that you will be able to not only improve your health but also help you to lose the weight that you want. With this in mind, it is likely that you are going to wonder what is going to make a healthy and nutritious diet for you to try out.

The first thing to add to your plate is plenty of vegetables and fruits. Fresh produce is always the best choice because it is going to give your body all the nutrients that it is looking to stay healthy. When you make your meals, you should rely on as many vegetables and fruits as you can. You also need to add a wide variety to your plate so that you get a variety of vitamins and minerals, rather than eating the same two or three products each time.

In addition, you should pick out some protein sources to help your muscles stay strong. There are many protein sources that you can choose, but some of these options are considered better than others. Lean options such as chicken, fish, turkey, and lean ground beef will work well. Having fatty meats on occasion, such as bacon, are fine as long as you limit these a little bit. Make sure to add some fish into your diet to make sure you get those healthy fats, and other healthy nutrients into your diet plan.

Dairy products are also supported on this diet plan, as long as you go with sources that do not have a lot of sugar added to them. Some options that are good include milk, yogurt, cheese, sour cream, cream cheese, and more. If you go with yogurt, make sure that you do not get the kinds that already have fruit and other things added in them. These usually contain a lot more sugar than regular yogurt. It is much better to get plain yogurt and add in your own fruit for some flavoring without all the sugar.

Carbs are just fine when you are on an intermittent fast and as long as you pick out some that are whole grain and good for the body, then you can consume them. If you are going on the ketogenic diet or something similar, you may be told to limit your carb consumption, but for those who are just doing intermittent fasting without the diet plan attached, it is fine to add in some healthy carbs to your meals.

Now that we have brought up the idea of eating carbs, we also need to explore the idea of being smart with the kinds of carbs that you consume. Do not go and eat a donut and assume that is what we meant and then get mad because it doesn't help you lose weight. When you are picking out carbs, you will want to pick out whole grain or whole wheat. These pack the most nutrients inside of them and won't fill you up on sugars, even if they are hidden, so you get the most out of this diet plan.

In addition to following some of the rules above, make sure that the diet you follow is varied. This is going to be the easiest way for you to add in a ton of nutrients to your body, and can also give you the health, the energy, and more than you are looking for while fasting. You are able to mix up the ingredients and the types of meals that you have to ensure that you get all of the variety.

Of course, it is fine to have a little cheat or something sweet on occasion. This diet is not as restrictive as some of the others and does allow for the occasional treat. As long as you know how to limit yourself and not take this too far, you are going to be fine when it comes to enjoying an indulgence on occasion.

More Than Fasting (tips to make it work)

Now we are on to the good part! We are going to take a look at some of the things that you need to try out to ensure that you are going to get the most out of your intermittent fast. There are a lot of people who are worried about going on this kind of fast because they worry that it will be too hard or that they will end up doing it the wrong way. But with the tips in this chapter, you will find that it is easier to get started on intermittent fasting than you would ever believe.

Pick the kind that works for you

Earlier in this guidebook, we talked about the fact that there are several different protocols that you can choose from when it comes to intermittent fasting. This may seem to make the fasting a bit more difficult to follow, but in fact, it makes it easier. Each person is able to choose the kind of fasting that works for them, the kind that will be easy enough for them to follow and the kind that will fit in with their schedule.

To see weight loss and health benefits, you do want to make sure that the protocol that you pick is going to be a bit difficult and adds in a little challenge for you. But outside of that, you can pick any of the protocols that you would like to help you get the best results. Whether this includes the 16/8 fast because it helps you to do a bit of fasting each day and keep on track, or the 24 hours fast because you have a few days a week where it is already hard to get a meal into your day or some other method, you will find that there is sure to be an option for you.

Eat healthier foods along the way

While on an intermittent fast, you can technically eat any kind of food that you would like. There really isn't a set diet plan that goes with this. But face the facts; if you want to lose weight and improve your health with intermittent fasting, it is not going to be enough to just limit the amount of time that you get to eat. You also need to make sure that the majority of the foods you consume are going to be healthy.

This is not as hard as it may seem in the beginning. If you are able to fill your plates up each meal with healthy fruits and vegetables, whole grains, lean meats, and some healthy fats, then you will be well on your way to seeing some great results when you fast.

Find someone to do it with you

Going on a fast on your own can seem like a lot of work, and like it is not going to be all that much fun either. You may worry that this is going to be too hard for you to work with at all, or that you are not going to see the results that you want because you have to watch everyone else eating whenever they want to. One of the best ways to make sure that you are going to get the results that you would like is to find a friend or a family member who is willing to go on the fast with you.

When you find someone who is willing and able to go on an intermittent fast with you, whether they follow the same protocol as you or not, you will find that fasting is much easier. You can share recipes together, motivate one another when it seems really hard to keep on track or you want to give in, share recipes, and just encourage one another to see the best results.

Fast during your busy times

One thing that you are going to notice when you get started on intermittent fasting is that you get to have a lot of the control on how this diet plan is going to work. You can pick and choose the starting times, the ending times, and even the days when you are going to go on a fast. While it is best to not have two fasting days right in a row, you get the freedom to make this work.

For example, if you are going to follow the 16/8 protocol and you find that mornings are super busy for you, skip breakfast and push your meals back so that you get to eat lunch and then a late supper instead. If you are doing the 24 hours fast, pick a day that is going to be super busy and decide what will be your fasting day so you get a chance to just focus on your work and be productive rather than having to worry about meals.

You get to have a lot of flexibility when it comes to fasting and when things start and end for you. And this is one of the reasons that you are going to love starting on this eating plan. You can move things around, and each week does not have to be exactly the same all of the time. There is a lot of freedom to make this work for you.

Do I need to consider the ketogenic diet?

As you are going through the information about the intermittent fasting online and maybe in other books, you may hear a bit about how the ketogenic diet goes along with it. Rest assured that you can pick out the diet plan that you like the best to help you with this. As long as it includes healthy foods and not a lot of processed or junk foods, you are going to be able to lose weight. You do not have to add in a diet plan that is as restrictive as the ketogenic diet along with the intermittent fast to get results.

With that said, there are a lot of people who love the ketogenic diet, and they find that adding the fasting to it helps them to really lose weight and fat quickly. If you want to see the results in no time, and you are interested in improving your health drastically then the ketogenic diet tied in with an intermittent fast may be the answer that you are looking with.

It is possible to use both of these diet plans together. Intermittent fasting is more about the times of day when you are going to eat and the ketogenic diet is the types of foods that you would eat during those time periods. You do not have to go on an intermittent fasting diet in order to lose weight with the ketogenic diet and many people find that the ketogenic diet is hard enough. But for those who would like to balance their blood sugars and who are worried about losing weight more efficiently, combining these two diet plans together can be great.

With intermittent fasting, you will limit the hours that you are able to eat. Instead of allowing yourself to spread your meals and your snacks all throughout the day, you will limit it to just a few hours. Many people will choose to only eat between ten and six and fit in their macronutrients into that time period. Others will take two or three days during the week (separated out) where they are not allowed to eat at all and will fit their nutrients into the other days of the week.

The point is that you are limiting the amount of time that you are able to eat, forcing you to think more about the foods you consume. You also get the benefit of more fat burning, and weight loss, when you go with intermittent fasting so it can be helpful while on the ketogenic diet any time that you hit a plateau with your weight loss.

During the times you are allowed to eat, you will need to stick with the macronutrients that we discussed above that are approved for the ketogenic diet. You will still stick with high fat, moderate protein, and low carb diet plan even while intermittent fasting. You will just need to be more careful about the times you eat those macronutrients, but otherwise, you can follow the ketogenic diet exactly the same.

You do not need to follow the ketogenic diet with an intermittent fast if you do not want to though. The decision is going to be completely up to you and what you are comfortable with. Maybe you want to lose weight and improve your health quickly so you through it on there to help. Or maybe you want to try out fasting first to see how it works and then add in the ketogenic diet later. Or it is perfectly fine if you decide to just do intermittent fasting and not worry about the ketogenic diet at all! It is just another option to consider trying out to see if it works for you!

Add in some exercise

If you want to see even more results when you start with this kind of eating plan, then you need to make sure that you add in some exercise. This doesn't have to be intense and you don't need to spend hours in the gym to get the results that you would like. But it does allow you a chance to get the heart pumping and to work out the muscles, and that is always something that is great.

There are different options that you are able to choose with exercise based on what you like the best. The three main types are going to include cardio, weight training, and stretching. If you are going to do cardio though, make sure that you do it during your eating window. The body during the fast is not going to be able to convert the nutrients that are leftover into fuel fast enough to help you keep up with an intense workout like this, so waiting until after you have been able to fuel up, or even at the beginning of your next fasting window, is often best.

Outside of this caution, you are able to enjoy a wide variety of workouts based on your own needs. You may find that weight lifting does really well with intermittent fasting, which is why a lot of people like to go on a protocol like the Warrior Diet when they want to really improve their strength and see what happens with that.

You can choose the kind of exercise that you would like to use. It is best if you are able to do a combination of weight lifting, cardio, and stretching to help out all the parts of the body. But any exercise that you are able to do and are willing to keep up with consistently, even if it starts out at just ten or fifteen minutes a day, will provide you with the results that you need.

Try to get plenty of nutrients into the body

Fasting is not going to harm your body. But it does make the bodywork a bit harder than it used to do. This means that you need to take in plenty of good nutrients to ensure that the body has what it needs even during the fasting period. For the most part, if you work hard at eating a diet that is balanced and full of lots of whole foods and variety, you will do just fine when it comes to providing your body with the nutrients that it needs.

Some people worry that it is going to be too hard to get in the nutrients that their bodies need during this time. They think that the eating window is just too short on some of these plans and that it will be impossible. But in reality, the way that you eat in the Western world is the wrong way and it is allowing you to have too much time to eat.

If you make sure that you eat a variety of healthy foods, you are going to get in all of the great nutrients that your body needs, even more than you did on the traditional American diet. If you are still worried about this though, consider taking a multi-vitamin when you first get started to ensure that all of your basis are covered.

Meal plan ahead of time

Another thing that you should consider doing to make this process work a bit better for you and to ensure that you are going to see the best results when you go on this kind of diet plan or eating plan, then you may want to consider going on a meal plan. This takes a bit of time, but it is really going to make your life on an intermittent fast easier.

Some people find that when they spend time preparing out their meals, and when they already know what meals they are going to have when the fast is over, it can make life easier. Think about how hungry you are going to be if you miss breakfast during one of your fasts, or if you end up going a whole day without eating. And if you are brand new to all of this, it is likely that you are going to have a bunch of cravings at the same time. If you have nothing planned to eat ahead of time, how likely do you think it is that you will reach for something healthy when the fast ends? Or are you more likely to reach for something that is full of sugar and carbs and will kill the cravings?

Meal planning makes life easier. When the fasting is done, and you have the meals already prepared, then you will be set to go. When you don't have to think about the foods that you have to eat or the meals that you need to prepare after a long fast, it just makes the process easier. You can just grab the meal and eat when your fasting is over, and then you are set!

There are a lot of benefits to meal planning ahead of time, and there are different methods that you are able to work with. You can choose to work with freezer meals and get a whole month done ahead of time. Most people find that they are best if they can prepare for a week at a time. You can get all of your meals done ahead of time, and you are set to make it all work for you!

Easy Recipes to Make Fasting Easier

The next thing that we can take a look at is some of the best recipes that you are able to work with. These recipes are meant to make your life easier overall. While there is not one diet plan that works with intermittent fasting, eating healthy and making sure there is a lot of variety in your meals, it is going to be easier to lose the weight and increase your health the way that you would like. Some of the best recipes that you are able to work with will include:

Breakfasts

Mexican Potato Hash and Eggs

What's inside:

Chopped cilantro (6 Tbsp.)
Pitted and cubed avocado (1)
Pepper Jack cheese (6 Tbsp.)
Eggs (6)
Pepper (.25 tsp.)
Salt (.5 tsp.)
Olive oil (2 Tbsp.)
Russet potatoes (3)

How to make:

Take the potatoes and peel and grate them. Drain out any of the liquid that is leftover.
Turn on your broiler. While that heats up, take out a skillet that is safe for the oven and heats up some oil inside.
Once the oil starts to shimmer, add in the grated potatoes. Cook these until they start to brown and all the way cooked through.
After ten more minutes, add the pepper and salt and then toss it around to combine.
When ready, you can use a spoon in order to make 6 wells in the potato hash. Crack an egg into your wineglass and pour into the well. Do this with the rest of the eggs.

Turn the heat down a bit and cook the eggs all the way through.

After another 12 minutes, take the lid from the skillet and sprinkle a bit of cheese on the eggs.

Add the skillet to the broiler to cook until the cheese has time to melt. Take out of the broiler after 2 minutes.

Bring out six plates and spoon one egg with some of the hash onto each plate. Top with some avocado and some cilantro before serving.

Cheese and Broccoli Muffins

What's inside:

Cheddar cheese (.75 c.)
Pepper
Salt (.5 tsp.)
Chopped scallions (3)
Almond milk (.5 c.)
Eggs (12)
Broccoli florets (2 c.)

How to make:

To start this recipe, turn on the oven and let it heat up to 350 degrees. Prepare some muffin tins and set to the side.
Bring out a pot and fill with an inch of water. Add in a steamer basket and place the broccoli inside.
Cover this and heat the broccoli inside for about five minutes to make it crisp. Move the broccoli to a cutting board and give it some time to cool down before slicing.
Bring out a big bowl and whisk together the pepper, salt, scallions, milk, and eggs. Add in the prepared broccoli and toss around to combine.
Spoon a bit of this into each of the muffin tin areas and top with a bit of cheese. Place into the oven to bake.

After 25 minutes, the muffins should be done, and you can take them out of the oven. After a bit, you can serve warm.

Chocolate Chip and Banana Waffles

What's inside:

Chocolate chips (.25 c.)
Baking soda (.5 tsp.)
Smooth almond butter (.5 c.)
Eggs (2)
Mashed ripe bananas (2)

How to make:

Take out your waffle iron and coat with some cooking spray.
Bring out your blender and add in the eggs, bananas, baking soda, and almond butter and blend until it is smooth.
Transfer this kind of batter over to a bowl and then slowly fold in the chocolate chips until smooth.
Pour a bit of the batter into the waffle iron and then cook for a few minutes on each side.
Move the finished waffle over to a plate and then finish with the rest of the batter before serving.

Yogurt Parfaits

What's inside:

Chopped almonds (.5 c.)
Nonfat Greek yogurt, vanilla (32 oz.)
Orange juice (.25 c.)
Peeled and diced kiwis (2)
Hulled and diced strawberries (1 c.)

How to make:

Bring out a bowl and place the kiwis and strawberries inside. Add in the orange juice and toss around to coat.
In four glasses, layer half a cup of yogurt and top with some of the fruit mixture.
Top this with a tablespoon of chopped almonds and then repeat for the second layer.
Serve this or place in the fridge covered for a few days.

Pear and Cinnamon Oatmeal

What's inside:

Honey (1 Tbsp.)
Diced pears (2)
Cinnamon (.75 tsp.)
Almond milk (2 c.)
Water (2 c.)
Steel cut oats (2 c.)

How to make:

Take out your slow cooker and coat the inside of it with some cooking spray.
When the slow cooker is done, you can spread the oats out on the bottom evenly.
Take out a bowl and whisk together the cinnamon, milk, and water. When those are combined, add in the pears and toss around to combine with the rest.
Pour this mixture over your oats and then set the slow cooker on a low setting.
Cook this for seven hours on the low setting. Once the oatmeal is cooked, stir in the honey and then serve.

Lunch Recipes

Mediterranean Salad

What's inside:

Olive oil (1 Tbsp>)
Kalamata olives (.33 c.)
Chopped red onion (.5)
Chopped red bell pepper (1)
Chopped plum tomatoes (2)
Hothouse cucumber, chopped (.66 c.)
Pepper
Salt
Juice from one lemon

How to make:

To start this recipe, bring out a bowl and add in the olives, onion, bell pepper, tomatoes, and cucumber.
Toss this around to combine well.
When that is done, add in the pepper, salt, lemon juice, and olive oil. Toss a bit to coat the vegetables before serving.

Coconut Curry Salmon

What's inside:

Salt (.5 tsp.)
Curry powder (.25 tsp.)
Coconut milk (.5 c.)
Water (.25 c.)
Zest and juice from two limes
Salmon (1.25 lbs.)
Olive oil (2 Tbsp.)
Coconut flakes (.5 c.)

How to make:

Bring out a pan or a skillet and toast the coconut for a few minutes so it has time to brown.
Use a paper towel in order to wipe out the pan before adding in the olive oil.
When the oil has had time to heat up and is shimmering, add in the salmon and sprinkle on the lime zest.
Add in the water and steam the fish for about ten minutes or until the fish is cooked through.
When the fish is done, you can move the salmon over to a serving platter. Add the pan to the heat and cook off the liquid that is in the pan still.
Now you can add in the salt, curry powder, coconut flakes, coconut milk, and lime juice.

Reduce the heat to a simmer at this time and then cook for a few minutes, making sure to stir the whole time.

Cut the fish up so it is in four pieces. Spoon some of the sauce on top of the fish and then serve warm.

Miso Glazed Tuna

What's inside:

Tuna steaks (4)
Brown sugar (2 Tbsp.)
Mirin (.33 c.)
Sake (.33 c.)
White miso (.33 c.)

How to make:

Turn on the oven and let it heat up to 300 degrees. While that is heating up, you can take out a baking dish and prepare with some cooking spray.
In a pan that is on some low heat, whisk together the brown sugar, mirin, sake, and miso. Whisk this until the sugar has had time to melt.
Pour the glaze into a bowl and then add the tuna inside. Turn it around to coat and then place into the fridge to marinate for some time.
After 30 minutes, you can take the fish out and place into your baking dish. Place into the oven and let it bake for some time.
After 12 minutes, the fish is going to be done. Take it out of the oven and serve warm.

Chicken Quesadillas

What's inside:

Monterey Jack cheese (1.5 c.)
Sliced jalapeno pepper (1)
Whole wheat tortillas (8)
Pepper
Salt (.25 tsp.)
Ground cumin (1.5 tsp.)
Chicken breast (1 lb.)
Olive oil (1 Tbsp.)

How to make:

To start this recipe, turn on the oven and give it time to heat up to 400 degrees. While that is heating up, take out two baking sheets and prepare with some cooking spray.
Now bring out a skillet and heat up the olive oil inside. When the oil is warm, add in the pieces of chicken and warm them through.
After two minutes, add in the cumin, salt, and pepper and toss around to coat well.
Coat one side of half the tortillas with some cooking spray and then add to the baking sheet. Divide the chicken between the two of these, top with some jalapeno peppers and the cheese, and then add in the other tortilla.

Place these into the oven to bake. After eight minutes, the tortillas should be done.
Take them from the oven and give them some time to cool down before slicing and enjoying.

Pesto Pasta with Chicken

What's inside:

Parmesan cheese (.25 c.)
Pepper
Salt
Halved cherry tomatoes (1 c.)
Pesto (.75 c.)
Leftover chicken (8 oz.)
Whole grain spaghetti (12 oz.)

How to make:

Take out a big pot and fill it with some water. Let the water boil before you add in the noodles and let them cook until they are done. Drain out the noodles and then place into a skillet.
Add the leftover chicken to this and then toss with the spaghetti to warm up.
Add in the pesto, tomatoes, pepper, and salt and cook for a bit longer, allowing the flavors to have some time to combine before moving on.
Move the pasta to a big bowl and then sprinkle with some cheese before serving.

Dinner Recipes

Sweet and Spicy Chicken Fingers

What's inside:

Sriracha (2 tsp.)
Honey (.5 c.)
Brown rice cereal (3 c.)
Pepper
Salt
Chicken breast tenders (1.25 lbs.)

How to make:

Turn on the oven and give it time to heat up to 375 degrees. While the oven is heating up, prepare a baking sheet with some cooking spray.
Sprinkle both sides of the chicken with some pepper and salt.
Place the brown rice cereal into a plastic bag and then use a rolling pin in order to crush it into some smaller pieces. When this is done, pour the cereal into a big bowl.
In another bowl, whisk together the sriracha and the honey.
Dip each of the tenders into the honey mixture and then let the extra drip off. Then dredge in the rice cereal, pressing it in evenly on all sides.

Add the chicken to the prepared baking sheet, making sure that there is some space left in between each side. Place into the oven.

After half an hour, the chicken is going to be done and you can serve warm.

Cilantro Lime Chicken

What's inside:

Olive oil (2 Tbsp.)
Cooking spray
Chicken thighs (1.25 lbs.)
Pepper
Salt
Red pepper flakes (.25 tsp.)
Brown sugar (1 Tbsp.)
Minced garlic cloves (2)
Cilantro, chopped (.33 c.)
Limes (3)

How to make:

Take two of the limes and zest and juice them. Slice up the third lime and set it aside. Bring out a small bowl and whisk together the lime juice and zest along with the pepper, salt, red pepper flakes, brown sugar, garlic, and cilantro.
Add in the chicken and toss it around to combine. Cover up the bowl and let it marinate for half an hour or longer before continuing.
At this time, you can turn on the oven and let it heat up to 350 degrees. Take out a baking dish and prepare it with some cooking spray.

While that is heating up, you can add some olive oil to a skillet and when the oil is hot, add in the chicken thighs and marinade and let them start to boil.

When a boil is reached, reduce the heat and cook the chicken until it has time to brown on both sides.

Move the sauce and the chicken over to your baking dish and add the slices of lime on top. Cover with some foil and add to the oven.

After 20 minutes, your chicken should be cooked through. Serve right away.

Chicken Enchilada Casserole

What's inside:

Corn tortillas (12)
Jarred salsa (2.5 c.)
Pepper
Salt
Black beans (1 can)
Chicken breast (8 oz.)
Cooking spray

How to make:

Turn on the oven to 350 degrees and while that is heating up, take a baking dish and coat it with some cooking spray.
Using a medium bowl, combine the black beans and the chicken. Toss with some pepper and salt.
Spread half a cup of salsa on the bottom of your baking dish and top with four of the tortillas.
Top with half the chicken, .75 cup of salsa, and half a cup of cheese. Repeat these layers ending with the cheese and then place into the oven.
After 40 minutes, the dish should be done. Take it out of the oven and give it some time to cool down before slicing and serving.

Easy Meatloaf

What's inside:

Pepper (.25 tsp.)
Salt (.5 tsp.)
Beaten egg (1)
Minced garlic clove (1)
Chopped onion (1)
Quick cooking oats (.75 c.)
BBQ sauce (1 c.)
Ground beef (1.5 lbs.)

How to make:

Turn on the oven and give it time to heat up to 350 degrees. Use some cooking spray to coat a loaf pan.
While the oven heats up, take out a big bowl and add together the pepper, salt, egg, garlic, onion, oats, half a cup of BBQ sauce and the beef.
Add this mixture to the prepared loaf pan and make it as level as possible. Pour the rest of the BBQ on top of the meatloaf and then put into the oven.
After an hour, check the internal temperature of the meat. When it reaches 155 degrees, you can take it out of the oven and give it some time to cool down.
Slice into eight pieces and enjoy.

Grilled Steak

What's inside:

Olive oil (2 Tbsp.)
Chopped scallions (2)
Drained capers (2 Tbsp.)
Cilantro leaves (1 c.)
Pepper
Salt
Sirloin steak (1.25 lbs.)
Minced garlic clove (1)
Juice from one lemon
Water (.25 c.)

How to make

Turn on the oven to 400 degrees. Prepare a grill pan or a skillet with some cooking spray.
Take the steak out and sprinkle both sides with the pepper and salt.
Heat up the grill pan over high heat and when it is hot, add in the steak. Cook on both sides for a few minutes to help roast it for a bit.
Place this skillet or pan into the oven and let it roast for a bit. When the steak reaches 145 degrees, which will take around 12 minutes, it is done.
Take the steak out of the oven and let it cool down for five minutes.

At this time, take out a blender and blend together the garlic, lemon juice, water, olive oil, scallions, capers, and cilantro. Blend to make it nice and smooth with a few chunks inside.

Slice up the steak thinly and then serve with your herb sauce.

Easy Snack Recipes

Spiced Popcorn

What's inside:

Cayenne pepper
Salt
Smoked paprika (.5 tsp.)
Onion powder (1 tsp.)
Garlic powder (1 tsp.)
Popcorn kernels (.5 c.)
Olive oil (3 Tbsp.)

How to make

Take out a pot and add a few tablespoons of oil to it. When the oil is warm, add in three of the popcorn kernels. When one starts to pop, you can add in the rest.
Cover up the pot and shake it around a few times to prevent the kernels from burning. Once they are all fully popped, move the popcorn over to a bowl.
Spray the popcorn using your cooking spray. Use clean hands to toss the cooking spray all over.
In another bowl mix together the cayenne, salt, paprika, onion powder, and garlic powder.

Sprinkle the spice mix on top of the popcorn and mix around until it is coated through before serving.

Snickerdoodle Pecans

What's inside:

Salt
Vanilla (.5 tsp.)
Ground cinnamon (.5 tsp.)
Maple syrup (2 Tbsp.)
Brown sugar (2 Tbsp.)
Raw pecans (1.5 c.)

How to make:

Turn on the oven and let it have time to heat up to 350 degrees. Bring out a baking sheet and add on some parchment paper.
In a bowl, add the pecans inside and top with the salt, vanilla, cinnamon, maple syrup, and brown sugar. Toss it around in order to coat evenly.
Spread the pecans in a single layer on your baking sheet and then add into the oven.
After 12 minutes, the pecans should be slightly browned and fragrant. Take out of the oven and serve warm.

Almond-Stuffed Dates

What's inside:

Pitted dates (20)
Almonds (20)

How to make

Take one almond and place it inside of a date.
Repeat this will all of the almonds and all of the dates. Serve at room temperature when you are ready.

Chocolate Chip Peanut Butter Energy Bites

What's inside:

Chocolate chips (.25 c.)
Honey (2 Tbsp.)
Vanilla (.5 tsp.)
Unsweetened coconut flakes (.5 c.)
Creamy peanut butter (.75 c.)
Old fashioned oats (1 c.)

How to make:

To start on this recipe, turn on the oven and give it time to heat up to 350 degrees. Prepare a baking sheet with some parchment paper.

Spread the oats onto a baking sheet and place this into the oven to bake. After 5 minutes, the oats are going to be browned and you can take them out of the oven to chill.

Bringing out a food processor, blend together the honey, vanilla, coconut, peanut butter, and oats until they are smooth.

Move this batter to a bowl and then fold in the chocolate chips. Spoon out some of the bathers into balls and put onto the baking sheet. Continue doing until all of the dough is gone.

Place these into the fridge to chill for 15 minutes or longer before serving.

No-Bake Granola Bars

What's inside:

Pumpkin seeds (2 Tbsp.)
Chopped raw almonds (2 Tbsp.)
Rolled oats (.75 c.)
Creamy almond butter (.75 c.)
Honey (.25 c.)
Pitted dates (1 c.)

How to make:

Take out a baking dish and line with some parchment paper and coat the paper with some cooking spray.
Take out the blender or food processor and add in the dates until they become almost like a paste.
Now add in the oats, almond butter, and honey and blend until it is all combined. Move this to a bowl.
Add in the pumpkin seeds and almonds and fold gently until it is combined.
Spoon this mixture into the prepared baking dish and then spread it out evenly while pushing it down.
Cover the dish with some plastic wrap and add to the fridge to set. This is going to take an hour or two to happen.

Take the bars out of the fridge and then slice into 8 bars, or however many you would like.
Wrap each of the individual bars in some plastic wrap and leave in the fridge until you need them.

The Routine

Each of the protocols that are available when you are on an intermittent fast is going to be a bit different. And though we did spend a bit of time looking at the answers to how each of these work, you will find that this can seem complicated until you get started. Using the recipes that we talked about above, we are going to take a look at the different options that are available based on the intermittent fasting protocol that you decide to go on!

The 16/8 protocol

The first example that we are going to look at when it comes to a meal plan with intermittent fasting is the 168 diet plan. This one is going to ask you to restrict the meals that you have to just 8 hours of the day. Instead of eating meals from the moment that you wake up until the moment you go to sleep, you will find just eight hours of the day that you are willing to eat within, and that is where all of your meals and snacks need to fall into.

This can be hard in the beginning, but it can also be as easy as cutting out breakfast or at least eating it late, and then making sure that you do not eat anything after you are done with supper. So no more early morning snacking and no more snacks or meals later in the night when it is almost time for bed. You can choose pretty much any time zone that you would like to work with when you are on this kind of fast, but the plan that we are going to take a look at will be eating between 10 in the morning and 6 in the evening. The plan that you are able to use to make this work includes:

Day 1:	Day 2:	Day 3:
10 AM: Mexican Potato Hash and Eggs 2 PM: Mediterranean Salad 6 PM: Sweet and Spicy Chicken Fingers	10 AM: Cheese and Broccoli Muffins 2 PM: Coconut Curry Salmon 6 PM: Cilantro Lime Chicken	10 AM: Chocolate Chip and Banana Waffles 2 PM: Miso Glazed Tuna 6 PM: Chicken Enchilada Casserole
Day 4: 10 AM: Yogurt Parfaits 2 PM: Chicken Quesadillas 6 PM: Easy Meatloaf	Day 5: 10 AM: Pear and Cinnamon Oatmeal 2 PM:: Pesto Pasta with Chicken 6 PM: Grilled Steak	

24 Hour Fast

The second protocol routine that we are going to take a look at here is the 24 hours fast. This is where you are going to spend 24 hours without eating anything except some water and black coffee if you need. This is a great way to really get the metabolism up and running and will help you to really limit the number of calories that you are consuming on a regular basis.

Now, you do not have to go a whole day without eating to get the benefits. With the routine that we are going to take a look at with this one will have us going from supper one day to supper the next day. But you can make this work for your needs. If you find that going from breakfast one day to breakfast the next day is going to work the best for you. As long as there are 24 hours between the two meals, it is going to work just fine.

In addition, just like you see with this routine, there needs to be a break between the fasts. You should not have two consecutive days where you are fasting for 24 hours. This can end up slowing the metabolism down too much and can reverse the benefits that you are looking for. But with a plan that has a few days in between, you will find that the 24 hour fast is going to be really effective for your health and weight loss goals. The routine that you are able to follow when going on a 24 hour fast will include:

Day 1:	Day 2:	Day 3:
10 AM: Mexican Potato Hash and Eggs 2 PM: Mediterranean Salad 6 PM: Sweet and Spicy Chicken Fingers	6 PM: Cilantro Lime Chicken	10 AM: Chocolate Chip and Banana Waffles 2 PM: Miso Glazed Tuna 6 PM: Chicken Enchilada Casserole
Day 4:	Day 5:	Day 6:
10 AM: Cheese and Broccoli Muffins 2 PM: Coconut Curry Salmon 6 PM: Grilled Steak	10 AM: Yogurt Parfaits 2 PM: Chicken Quesadillas 6 PM: Easy Meatloaf	6 PM: Pesto Pasta with Chicken

Warrior Diet

The next protocol that we are going to take a look at is the Warrior diet. This is going to be similar to what we see with the 16/8 protocol, but we are going to limit the amount of time that you get to eat from eight hours to just four hours. In this time period, there is usually only enough time to eat a few meals throughout the day. This can seem hard to work with sometimes, but you will find that it can really get the metabolism to speed up, and will do some wonders for helping you to restrict the amount of calories that you are consuming on a regular basis.

This one can be a little bit unique to work with, and often it is best if you are able to start with one of the other protocols and then build up a bit to this one over time. The routine that you are able to work on if you would like to try out the Warrior diet will include the following?

Day 1:	Day 2:	Day 3:
2 PM: Mediterranean Salad	2 PM: Miso Glazed Tuna	2 PM: Chocolate Chip and

6 PM: Sweet and Spicy Chicken Fingers	6 PM: Chicken Enchilada Casserole	Banana Waffles 6 PM: Pesto Pasta with Chicken
Day 4: 2 PM: Coconut Curry Salmon 6 PM: Grilled Steak	Day 5: 2 PM: Chicken Quesadillas 6 PM: Easy Meatloaf	

In addition to these times and meals, you are welcome to enjoy some snacks along the way. Just make sure that you are able to get them in so that they fall within your time frames for the diet plan that you are working with. Make sure that you try out some of the different options that we have prepared for you in the previous section to help you to get the best snacks possible while on an intermittent fast!

Chapter 9: The Potential Downsides of Intermittent Fasting

While there are a lot of benefits that come with intermittent fasting, it is important to also realize that there are going to be a few downsides that we need to watch out for as well. Some side effects are going to pop up in the beginning as your body makes adjustments from eating all of the time to finding that it is more limited to eating only during certain times. Some of the side effects that you need to watch out for are:

Withdrawal

Withdrawal is something that is going to happen when the body starts to lack some of the substances that it had in the past, substances that it has become addicted to. When most of us are going to think about withdrawal, we are going to think more about drug abuse and abuse of alcohol. Sure, these are going to be examples of this, but you can also have the signs of withdrawal to other things as well. Often it is going to be from a lack of sugar and carbs being constantly supplied to the body.

This can be a positive thing because it shows us that the body is ridding itself of the toxic substances that were inside. But it is not going to feel that great. You may feel grouchy, tired, and like everything is going to irritate you all of the time. If you notice that the symptoms are starting to get worse in the process, and you feel shaky, like fainting, and more, then it may be time to seek some professional help.

Anxiety attacks

Another side effect that you may deal with when it comes to intermittent fasting is that you may have some anxiety attacks. This is going to happen when you end up going for a longer period of time without food and can be more likely if you have never gone on a fast and then do some of the longer fasts right away. This anxiety attack can sometimes happen when you feel like you are not getting enough nutrition into the body.

Find some breathing exercises that you are able to use to help you get through some of the anxiety that you are feeling. If you let the anxiety get to you, then it is more likely that you are going to binge eat or give up on your fast before it is time. And the more often that it happens, the harder it is going to be to get the results that are promised with this kind of fasting.

The distress of the stomach.

Since you will find that going on an intermittent fast does include some detoxing, it is possible that during the first few times that you do it, there could be some digestive distress that goes on. This is because the body is trying to flush out a lot of the residual matter that is found there, along with getting rid of whatever may have been stuck in there for a long period of time. As long as it is just a bit of discomfort in the stomach during this time, it is nothing to really worry about.

At times though, this can get worse, and you need to be aware of that. If you find that the symptoms of this are not going away, then it is time to seek some medical attention to help you.

Sometimes you are going to find that this kind of distress will include cramping, pain, and discomfort. If you have never gone on a fast before then this is pretty common. They may occur when the acids in the stomach are starting to irritate the walls of your stomach. If the pain gets too severe to handle in this case, then it may be time to readjust some of your eating windows and take the fasting a bit slower to figure out what works the best for you.

Headaches

This is often a signal that you are going through withdrawal, although it is possible that you will deal with the headaches without some of the other symptoms that we talked about before. This is going to be a natural reaction that occurs in the brain when you suddenly change up the chemical composition through the detox process of intermittent fasting. You may find that you get a slight headache but it goes away on its own. You can also take some Tylenol or Aspirin to help out with these headaches if they get a bit too much to bear.

Pre-existing conditions

Another thing that we need to watch out for in this eating plan is the idea of having a condition for your health before you start on the plan. Some conditions are not going to fare well when it comes to fasting, and it is important to really watch out for this and be aware that it could be a major problem.

For example, hypoglycemia is going to be a condition which is uncomfortable and triggered when we have low blood sugar. It can be aggravated quite a bit when you go through a period of fasting that is longer than just when you sleep at night. While this condition is not usually going to be life-threatening, it can cause a reaction that is a bit more serious and can get worse when the sufferer goes on a fast that lasts too long. They could start to lose their consciousness and they are not able to function the way that they should.

If you already have a pre-existing health issue that you are working with, make sure that you discuss going on an intermittent fast with your doctor ahead of time. This will help you to prepare and do the fast in a manner that is going to work the best for your condition.

Diabetes

For many diabetics, it is going to be necessary to take some medications in order to help you to feel better. And most diabetics are going to ask you to go on a strict diet to help make sure that the condition is under control as much as possible. This could include doing things like eating so many times each day, limiting carb and sugar consumption, and drinking lots of water.

In most cases, intermittent fasting is not going to be recommended when you are a diabetic. It does depend on your condition and it doesn't hurt to talk to your doctor about it to see what they say about going on this eating plan and if it is something that you should try out or not.

Flu-Like Symptoms

One thing that some people are going to notice when they go on an intermittent fast is that they are going to feel like they are being hit hard by the flu. This is even truer if you decide to go on a ketogenic diet along with it. This is because you will find that your body is not going to be used to not having these steady stream of carbs cut out by so much, and you are going to go through some signs of withdrawal that can be unpleasant.

You will find that these symptoms are going to be severe and hard to get through for a bit. You are going to feel weak, have headaches, and feel like you are going through a flue that can make things difficult. And if the cravings end up finding you during this time as well, that is just going to make the situation that much worse. You are going to want to crave things during your fasting time, and giving in is going to make it difficult for you to get the results that you want.

The good news here is that with a bit of practice, and with just bearing through it for a week or so of the fasting, you will start to feel better. This is just a response to the body not being used to a lack of carbs and food all of the time. it is going to learn how to adjust fairly quickly, and then you will be able to get through the fast without feeling bad, and while still getting more energy, mental clarity, and the other benefits you are looking for on the fast.

Pregnancy and nursing

While pregnancy is not a condition that will count like the others, it is one that you need to consider when you go on an intermittent fast. You should not go on this eating plan if you are pregnant or nursing. This is because you need much more nutrients when you are pregnant and nursing, and you need to have them spread out more through the day compared to what you are going to see with fasting. It is definitely not recommended to go on a full day fast when you are in this condition.

If you are dealing with morning sickness and you have trouble eating on regular intervals, this is usually not a big deal and is pretty normal during pregnancy. As long as the baby is getting the nutrients and is growing like normal, then you will not have to worry about this as much.

There are a few concerns that you need to keep in mind when it comes to working with intermittent fasting and getting it to work for you. Most of these are just going to be temporary and are not going to be a big deal over time. Once you adjust to the eating plan and get used to the idea that you are not allowed to eat all of the time, you will find that you are going to feel so much better on this diet plan and want to stick with it for the long term.

Conclusion

Thank for making it through to the end of *Intermittent Fasting for the Body and Mind* let's hope it was informative and able to provide you with all of the tools you need to achieve your goals whatever they may be.

The next step is to start implementing intermittent fasting into your life. Whether you are overweight, a normal weight, or obese and you want to get your health under control, you will find that you are able to benefit when it comes to working with an intermittent fast. This is a great way to ensure that you are eating foods that are healthy and wholesome for you and can make it so much easier or you to maintain or lose weight than any other plan out there.

This guidebook has taken some time to discuss some of the negatives that come with being obese. Many of these are things that we already know, but we often choose to ignore them, which is made evident when we take a look at the rising epidemic of obesity in our country and how it is likely to continue growing more and more in the future.

While there are a lot of different methods out there that promise they will help you to control your weight and even to help you lose a lot of weight quickly, none are going to work as well or be as efficient as what we are able to see when it comes to intermittent fasting. And that is why we spent so much time exploring fasting and how it can work to make things easier for you!

When you are ready to fight obesity and lose weight in a natural and healthy way, and in a manner that you are likely to be able to maintain for the long term, make sure to check out this guidebook and learn how you can use intermittent fasting to help you get it all done.

Finally, if you found this book useful in any way, a review on Amazon is always appreciated!

Sources

1. https://www.dietdoctor.com/intermittent-fasting
2. https://www.healthline.com/nutrition/intermittent-fasting-guide
3. https://www.nerdfitness.com/blog/a-beginners-guide-to-intermittent-fasting/
4. https://www.sciencedirect.com/science/article/pii/S193152441400200X
5. https://ibima.org/
6. https://www.ncbi.nlm.nih.gov/pmc/articles/PMC3946160/
7. https://www.ncbi.nlm.nih.gov/pmc/articles/PMC3946160/
8. https://www.ncbi.nlm.nih.gov/pmc/articles/PMC329619/
9. https://www.ncbi.nlm.nih.gov/pubmed/1548337
10. https://www.ncbi.nlm.nih.gov/pubmed/12425705
11. https://www.ncbi.nlm.nih.gov/pmc/articles/PMC3106288/
12. https://www.ncbi.nlm.nih.gov/pubmed/24048020
13. https://www.ncbi.nlm.nih.gov/pubmed/2405717
14. https://www.ncbi.nlm.nih.gov/pubmed/25540982

15. https://www.ncbi.nlm.nih.gov/pubmed/3245934
16. https://www.ncbi.nlm.nih.gov/pubmed/15833943
17. https://jamesclear.com/the-beginners-guide-to-intermittent-fasting
18. https://www.health.harvard.edu/blog/intermittent-fasting-surprising-update-2018062914156
19. https://www.healthline.com/nutrition/10-health-benefits-of-intermittent-fasting#section1
20. https://www.eatthis.com/intermittent-fasting-benefits/
21. https://www.healthline.com/nutrition/6-proven-ways-to-lose-belly-fat
22. https://www.sciencedirect.com/science/article/pii/S193152441400200X

www.ingramcontent.com/pod-product-compliance
Lightning Source LLC
Chambersburg PA
CBHW021823170526
45157CB00007B/2666